DECOMPRESSIVE TECHNIQUES

Other books in this series

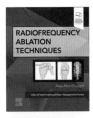 Alaa Abd-Elsayed, Radiofrequency Ablation Techniques, 1e
ISBN: 9780323870634

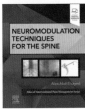 Alaa Abd-Elsayed, Neuromodulation Techniques for the Spine, 1e
ISBN: 9780323875844

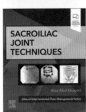 Alaa Abd-Elsayed, Sacroiliac Joint Techniques, 1e
ISBN: 9780323877541

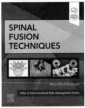 Alaa Abd-Elsayed, Spinal Fusion Techniques, 1e
ISBN: 9780323882231

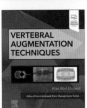 Alaa Abd-Elsayed, Vertebral Augmentation Techniques, 1e
ISBN: 9780323882262

DECOMPRESSIVE TECHNIQUES

Atlas of Interventional Pain Management Series

Alaa Abd-Elsayed, MD, MPH, CPE, FASA

Medical Director, UW Health Pain Services
Medical Director, UW Pain Clinic
Division Chief, Chronic Pain Management
Department of Anesthesiology
University of Wisconsin
Madison, Wisconsin
United States

ELSEVIER

Elsevier
1600 John F. Kennedy Blvd.
Ste 1800
Philadelphia, PA 19103-2899

DECOMPRESSIVE TECHNIQUES
Atlas of Interventional Pain Management Series

ISBN: 978-0-323-87751-0

Senior Content Development Manager: Somodatta Roy Choudhury
Executive Content Strategist: Michael Houston[†]
Senior Content Development Specialist: Malvika Shah
Publishing Services Manager: Shereen Jameel
Project Manager: Maria Shalini
Senior Designer: Patrick C. Ferguson

Printed in India.

Last digit is the print number: 9 8 7 6 5 4 3 2 1

Dedication

I would like to dedicate this book to my parents,
my wife, and my two beautiful kids, Maro and George.

Contributors

Hamid R. Abbasi, MD, PhD
Chief Medical Officer, Inspired Spine
Burnsville, Minnesota
United States

Alaa Abd-Elsayed, MD, MPH, CPE, FASA
Medical Director, UW Health Pain Services
Medical Director, UW Pain Clinic
Division Chief, Chronic Pain Management
Department of Anesthesiology
University of Wisconsin
Madison, Wisconsin
United States

Rohit Aiyer, MD
Richmond Interventional Pain Management
Staten Island, New York
United States

Ryan Budwany, MD, MPH, MBA
Director of Pain Medicine
CAMC Teays Valley Hospital
Spine and Nerve Centers of the Virginias
Hurricane, West Virginia
United States

Alyson Engle, MD
Assistant Professor
Division of Pain Medicine
Department of Anesthesiology
Northwestern University Feinberg School of Medicine
Chicago, Illinois
United States

Nasir Hussain, MD, MSc
Assistant Professor
Anesthesiology
The Ohio State University, Wexner Medical Center
Columbus, Ohio
United States

Maher Kodsy, MD, MBA
Chairperson
Department of Anesthesiology
University Hospitals Elyria Medical Center
Elyria, Ohio
United States

Physician Director, Perioperative Services
Surgery
University Hospitals Elyria Medical Center
Elyria, Ohio
United States

President
Elyria Anesthesia Services, Inc.
Elyria, Ohio
United States

Merna Naji, MD
Physical Medicine and Rehabilitation
University of Pittsburgh Medical Center
Pittsburgh, Pennsylvania
United States

Yeshvant A. Navalgund, MD
Assistant Professor
Anesthesiology/Pain Medicine
West Virginia University
Morgantown, West Virginia
United States

Alopi M. Patel, MD
Assistant Professor
Department of Anesthesiology
Mount Sinai Morningside and West Hospital Center
New York, New York
United States

Christopher Robinson, MD, PhD
Anesthesiology & Interventional Chronic Pain
Beth Israel Deaconess Medical Center
Massachusetts
United States

Alexander J. Schupper, MD
Neurological Surgery
Mount Sinai Health System
New York, New York
United States

Jarod Speer, MD
The Ohio State University
Anesthesiology
Wexner Medical Center
Columbus, Ohio
United States

Jeremy M. Steinberger, MD
Assistant Professor
Neurosurgery & Orthopedics & Rehabilitation Medicine
Icahn School of Medicine at Mount Sinai
New York
United States

Nicholas R. Storlie, MD
Creighton University School of Medicine
Omaha, Nebraska
United States

Marianne Tanios, MD, MPH
Metro Health
Cleveland Clinic
Cleveland, Ohio
United States

Preface

Atlas of Interventional Pain Management Series provides indications for and describes techniques associated with advanced interventional pain management and decompression procedures.

The field of interventional pain medicine has progressed significantly in the past decade. Interventional pain physicians previously performed simple procedures and injections that both alleviated pain and eradicated the impetus for the noxious stimuli. Advanced procedures are now available to providers and patients that address painful conditions that were previously not amenable to intervention.

The *Atlas* series represents a landmark milestone in the published pain literature, as it provides a comprehensive guide to all currently available advanced pain procedures.

This *Atlas* title, *Decompressive Techniques*, discusses the critical topics of foraminotomy, discectomy, laminotomy, and more. Knowledge of the anatomy, patient selection, procedure techniques and strategies to optimize performance, and perioperative management is essential to the safe and successful performance of these procedures.

I would like to thank the authors for their original contributions. All chapters were written by experts in the field, and I am very grateful for the time they dedicated to crafting chapters that resonate with readers and offer top-quality content.

I also would like to thank the publisher for sponsoring this book and making it available for learners.

Alaa Abd-Elsayed, MD, MPH, CPE, FASA

Contents

Chapter 1

An Overview on the Anatomy of the Spine

Rohit Aiyer

Cervical Spine

The cervical spine is composed of seven vertebrae, with the first two vertebrae known as the atlas (C1) and axis (C2). The atlas contains a thick anterior arch and a thin posterior arch, which is ring-shaped and supports the cranium. The transverse process contains a transverse foramen, through which the artery passes. The vertebral foramen is large in diameter and contains the spinal cord which passes through. There are two arches: posterior and anterior. The anterior arch extends into the two lateral masses that articulate with the occipital condyles and inferior joint facets (Fig. 1.1). The posterior arch is comparatively

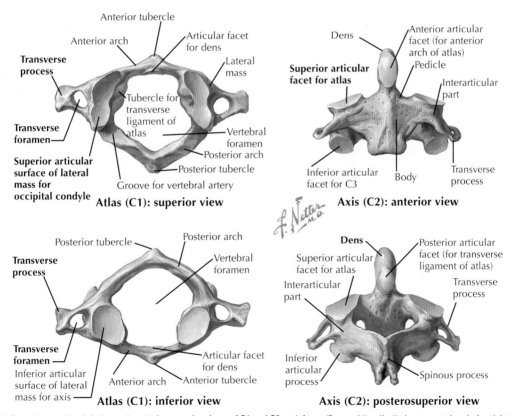

Fig. 1.1 Superior, anterior, inferior, and posterior-superior views of C1 and C2 vertebrae. (Source: https://netterimages.com/cervical-vertebrae-atlas-and-axis-labeled-rubin-general-anatomy-frank-h-netter-60487.html.)

thinner than the anterior arch and composes the posterior section of the lateral masses.

The body of the axis, C2, is fused to the body of the atlas to form the odontoid process, alternatively called the dens. Similar to the atlas, the transverse process of the axis contains two transverse foramen to allow for passage of the vertebral arteries (see Fig. 1.1). Unlike the atlas, the axis has a distinct bifid spinous process, which is formed from two laminae. The atlas and axis articulate between the superior facets of the axis with the inferior articular facet of the atlas, and the inferior articular facets of the axis articulate with the superior articular facets of the third cervical vertebra.[1] Compared with the atlas, the axis has a prominent superior process, does not contain tubercles on the transverse processes, and has a prominent spinous process.

The third to sixth cervical vertebrae (C3–C6) are anatomically similar to each other and different from the atlas and axis. The vertebral bodies are relatively small, and taller on the posterior aspect compared with the anterior part of the body (Fig. 1.2). The joints are formed through the articulation of two uncinate processes upward with the lower parts of the upper vertebrae to compose the uncovertebral joints, alternatively known as the Luschka joints.[1] The distance between the uncinate processes increases gradually descending from C3. The spinous processes at these levels are short and bifid, and protrude posteriorly and inferiorly (see Fig. 1.2). The vertebral artery runs transversely through the cervical vertebrae, lateral to the vertebral bodies and medial to the tubercles.

The body of the seventh cervical vertebra, C7, is unique in its appearance as the lateral mass is more elongated in the superior–inferior direction and thinner in the anteroposterior direction.[2] The spinous process of C7 is large and is not bifid, like the levels above.

The cervical spine has two longitudinal ligaments: anterior and posterior. The anterior longitudinal ligament is attached to the vertebral bodies, whereas the posterior longitudinal ligament is attached to the intervertebral disc (Fig. 1.3). The ligaments are utilized as stabilizers for the joints in the cervical spine.

Cervical Vertebrae

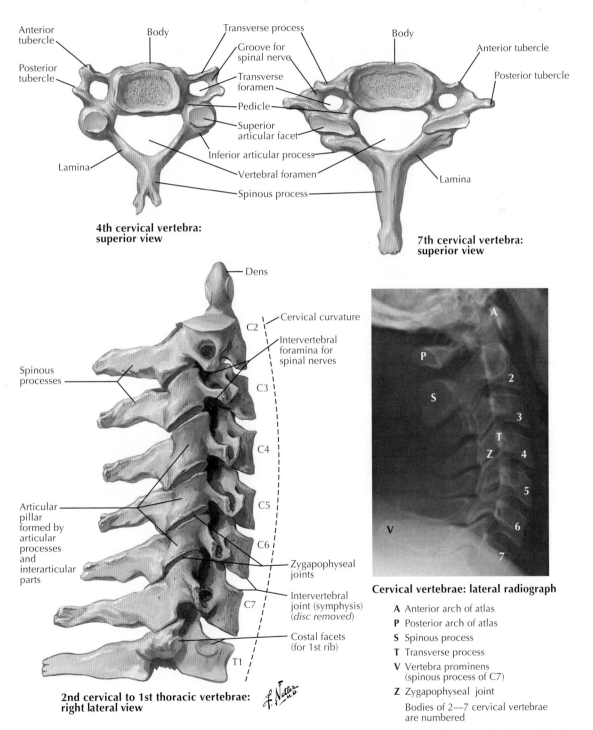

4th cervical vertebra: superior view

- Anterior tubercle
- Body
- Transverse process
- Groove for spinal nerve
- Posterior tubercle
- Transverse foramen
- Pedicle
- Superior articular facet
- Inferior articular process
- Lamina
- Vertebral foramen
- Spinous process

7th cervical vertebra: superior view

- Body
- Anterior tubercle
- Posterior tubercle
- Lamina

2nd cervical to 1st thoracic vertebrae: right lateral view

- Dens
- Cervical curvature
- C2
- Intervertebral foramina for spinal nerves
- Spinous processes
- C3
- C4
- C5
- Articular pillar formed by articular processes and interarticular parts
- C6
- Zygapophyseal joints
- C7
- Intervertebral joint (symphysis) (*disc removed*)
- Costal facets (for 1st rib)
- T1

Cervical vertebrae: lateral radiograph

- **A** Anterior arch of atlas
- **P** Posterior arch of atlas
- **S** Spinous process
- **T** Transverse process
- **V** Vertebra prominens (spinous process of C7)
- **Z** Zygapophyseal joint

  Bodies of 2—7 cervical vertebrae are numbered

Fig. 1.2 Sagittal and axial view of cervical vertebrae. (Source: https://netterimages.com/cervical-vertebrae-labeled-anatomy-atlas-3e-general-anatomy-frank-h-netter-4528.html.)

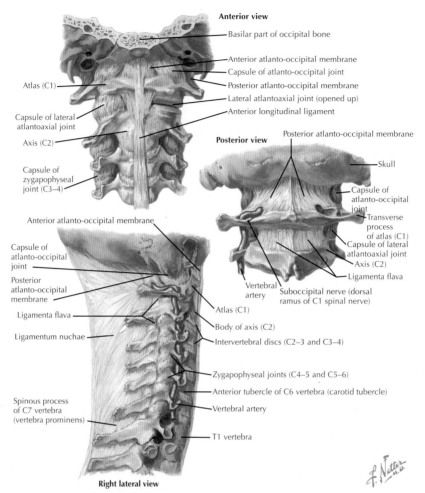

Fig. 1.3 Anterior, posterior and right lateral views of cervical vertebrae. (Source: https://www.netterimages.com/external-craniocervical-ligaments-unlabeled-general-anatomy-frank-h-netter-1323.html.)

There are six intervertebral cervical discs, with the first one located between C2 and C3. The disc is composed of four parts: nucleus pulposus, annulus fibrosus, and two cartilaginous endplates.[1] In the cervical spine, the anterior portion of the disc is thicker (by roughly one-third), and the annulus fibrosus is thicker in the posterior section (compared with the lumbar spine), which results in this part of the spine having a lordotic curve.[1] When the cervical disc has a protrusion or extrusion, it can cause stenosis, or narrowing of the spinal cord (Fig. 1.4).

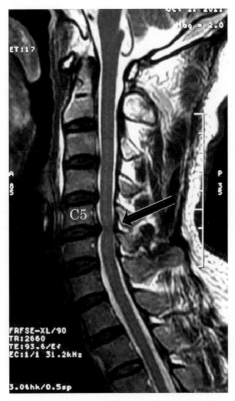

Fig. 1.4 Sagittal view of MRI cervical spine illustrating stenosis at C5–C6 level. (Source: https://www.journaloforthopaedicscience.com/article/S0949-2658(16)30176-2/abstract.)

Thoracic Spine

The thoracic spine is composed of 12 vertebrae. The vertebral bodies increase in size from superior to inferior. Anatomically, a thoracic vertebra consists of a vertebral arch, vertebral body, and seven processes. The body is composed of trabecular bone and is surrounded by a compact bone. The arch consists of bilateral pedicles and bilateral lamina, which connect the transverse and spinous processes. There are two inferior and two superior processes, comprising a total of four processes that articulate with adjacent processes.[3] This joint is known as a facet or zygapophyseal joint, which is where the inferior and superior facets meet (Fig. 1.5). Two symmetrical transverse processes project laterally from the vertebral arch, and the spinous process projects inferiorly and posteriorly from the vertebral arch.[3] When the thoracic vertebrae are aligned together, they produce a kyphotic curve (Fig. 1.6).

Thoracic vertebrae contain six costal facets per vertebra: two on the transverse process and four demifacets. The facets located on the transverse processes articulate with the rib, whereas the superior demifacet of an inferior vertebra articulates with the head of the rib that articulates with the inferior demifacet of a superior rib.[3] In addition, the vertebrae in this region have superior articular facets that face a posterolateral direction, the spinous processes are long, and protrude in a posteroinferior direction.[3]

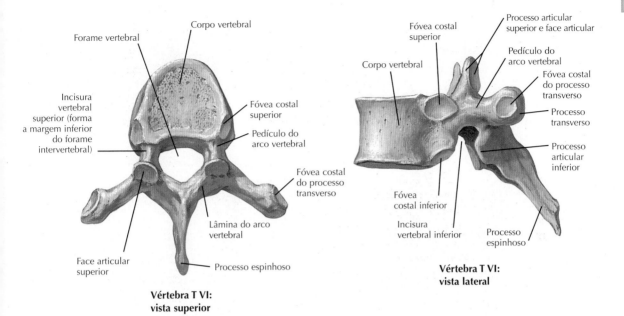

Forame vertebral

Corpo vertebral

Incisura
vertebral
superior (forma
a margem inferior
do forame
intervertebral)

Fóvea costal
superior

Pedículo do
arco vertebral

Fóvea costal
do processo
transverso

Lâmina do arco
vertebral

Face articular
superior

Processo espinhoso

**Vértebra T VI:
vista superior**

Fóvea costal
superior

Corpo vertebral

Processo articular
superior e face articular

Pedículo do
arco vertebral

Fóvea costal
do processo
transverso

Processo
transverso

Processo
articular
inferior

Fóvea
costal inferior

Incisura
vertebral inferior

Processo
espinhoso

**Vértebra T VI:
vista lateral**

Canal vertebral

Processo articular superior
e face articular

7ª costela

TVII

TVIII

TIX

Lâmina do
arco vertebral

Processo espinhoso da
vértebra T VII

Processo transverso da
vértebra T IX

Processo articular inferior (T IX)

Processo espinhoso (T IX)

**Vértebras T VII, T VIII e T IX:
vista posterior**

Corpo vertebral

Processo articular
superior e face
articular

Processo
transverso

Fóvea costal

Processo articular
inferior e face articular

Processo
espinhoso

**Vértebra T XII:
vista lateral**

Fig. 1.5 **Superior, posterior, and lateral view of thoracic vertebrae.** (Source: From Netter, FH. *Atlas of Human Anatomy*. 4th ed. Plate 154; Saunders: Philadelphia; 2006.)

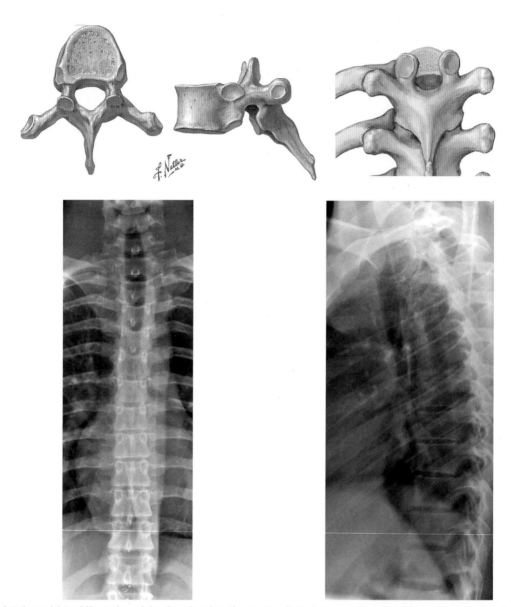

Fig. 1.6 Anterior and lateral X-ray view of the thoracic spine. (Source: https://netterimages.com/thoracic-vertebrae-unlabeled-radiography-frank-h-netter-61673.html.)

Lumbar Spine

The lumbar spine consists of five vertebrae that are larger than the vertebrae in the thoracic and cervical spine. Their large body surface area allows them to absorb axial forces from the entire body, including the head, neck, and trunk.[4] The formation of these five vertebrae allows for a concave curvature that is called a lumbar lordotic curve. Each vertebra consists of a vertebral body, vertebral arch, and seven processes.[5] The bodies of the vertebrae increase in size as they descend toward the coccyx. The arch combines with the posterior part of the body to form the spinal canal.[4] The arch is made up of bilateral pedicles that connect the body to the arch, and bilateral lamina that connect the transverse and spinous processes (Fig. 1.7). There are two sets of articular processes, two inferior and two superior, that connect the inferior and superior articular processes of adjacent vertebrae, respectively.[5] The facet or zygapophyseal joint is the anatomical location where the superior and inferior articular facets connect. The spinous process projects posteriorly and inferiorly from the vertebral arch. Finally, the two transverse processes project laterally from the arch, and is a point of contact for attachment of muscles and ligaments.[5] When there is enlargement or arthritis of the facet joint, this can lead to lumbar spinal stenosis, or narrowing of the spinal canal (Fig. 1.8). This can occur at one level, or sometimes in several levels along the lumbar spine (Fig. 1.9). The pars interarticularis should be noted as this is the anatomical area of the lamina located between the inferior and superior articular process and is important as this area is higher risk for development of spondylolysis (a stress fracture).

The lumbar disc contains two parts: fibrous annulus fibrosus (outer layer) and gelatinous nucleus pulposus (inner layer). The function is for absorption of axial forces. There are an anterior and a posterior longitudinal ligament, which connect to the vertebral body. The anterior ligament helps resist rotation, translation, and lumbar extension, whereas the posterior ligament resists flexion.[5]

The spinal cord runs through the center of the vertebral column and terminates at the conus medullaris, roughly at the level of L1–L2,[4] and the cauda equina, a bundle of spinal nerve roots runs from the termination of the spinal cord through to the remaining portion of the spinal canal. The coccyx consists of a trabecular bone that contains red marrow and is surrounded by compact bone.

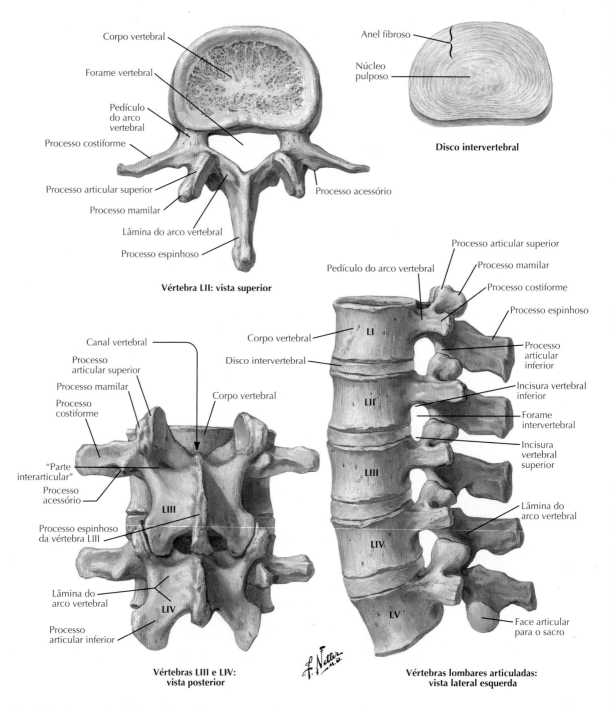

Corpo vertebral

Forame vertebral

Pedículo do arco vertebral

Processo costiforme

Processo articular superior

Processo mamilar

Lâmina do arco vertebral

Processo espinhoso

Processo acessório

Vértebra LII: vista superior

Anel fibroso

Núcleo pulposo

Disco intervertebral

Canal vertebral

Processo articular superior

Processo mamilar

Processo costiforme

"Parte interarticular"

Processo acessório

Processo espinhoso da vértebra LIII

Lâmina do arco vertebral

Processo articular inferior

Corpo vertebral

LIII

LIV

Vértebras LIII e LIV: vista posterior

Pedículo do arco vertebral

Corpo vertebral

Disco intervertebral

LI

LII

LIII

LIV

LV

Processo articular superior

Processo mamilar

Processo costiforme

Processo espinhoso

Processo articular inferior

Incisura vertebral inferior

Forame intervertebral

Incisura vertebral superior

Lâmina do arco vertebral

Face articular para o sacro

Vértebras lombares articuladas: vista lateral esquerda

Fig. 1.7 Superior, posterior, and lateral view of lumbar vertebrae. (Source: https://www.netterimages.com/lumbar-vertebrae-and-intervertebral-discspine-osteology-unlabeled-orthopaedics-frank-h-netter-1438.html.)

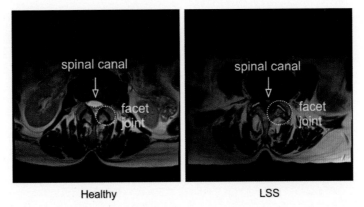

Fig. 1.8 MRI axial image of lumbar spine comparing healthy spine with a spine that has lumbar spinal stenosis *(LSS)*. (Source: https://www.oarsijournal.com/article/S1063-4584(14)00673-6/fulltext.)

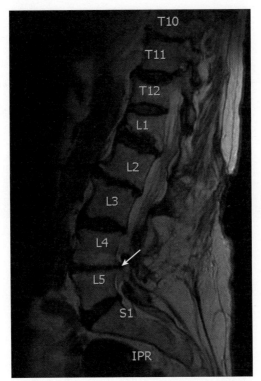

Fig. 1.9 MRI sagittal view of lumbar spine illustrating multilevel central canal stenosis in the lumbar spine. (Source: https://www.rheumatic.theclinics.com/article/S0889-857X(18)30033-4/fulltext.)

REFERENCES

1. Ombregt L. *A System of Orthopedic Medicine*. 3rd ed. London, England: Elsevier; 2013.
2. Kim DH, Henn JS, Vaccaro AR, Dickman CA. *Surgical Anatomy & Techniques to the Spine*. Philadelphia: Elsevier; 2006.
3. Waxenbaum JA, Reddy V, Futterman B. *Anatomy, Back, Thoracic Vertebrae*. Treasure Island (FL): StatPearls Publishing; 2021.
4. Sassack B, Carrier JD. *Anatomy, Back, Lumbar Spine*. Treasure Island (FL): StatPearls Publishing; 2021.
5. Waxenbaum JA, Reddy V, Williams C, Futterman B. *Anatomy, Back, Lumbar Vertebrae*. Treasure Island (FL): StatPearls Publishing; 2021.

Chapter 2

Surgical Instruments

Alexander J. Schupper, Jeremy M. Steinberger, and Alopi M. Patel

Introduction

Surgical decompression is the main objective for many spinal procedures. Decompression may be performed in the cervical, thoracic, lumbar, or sacral spine, from a single approach or a combination of anterior, lateral, or posterior approaches.[1] Traditionally, an open surgical technique has been utilized, however, minimally invasive spine (MIS) surgery techniques have gained traction due to improved perioperative morbidity, faster return to work, decreased cost, decreased opioid use, and decreased length of hospital stay. In this chapter, surgical instruments used in decompressive procedures of the spine will be introduced.

Cervical Approaches

ANTERIOR APPROACH VIA ANTERIOR CERVICAL DISCECTOMY AND FUSION (ACDF) OR ARTHROPLASTY

A scalpel is used for the skin incision (No. 10 or 15 blade) (Fig. 2.1) and subplatysmal dissection is performed with Metzenbaum scissors and non-toothed forceps. Medial structures (trachea and esophagus) are retracted using Cloward retractors, and blunt dissection exposes the prevertebral fascia. Dissection of the longus colli muscles is accomplished with electrocautery (Fig. 2.2).

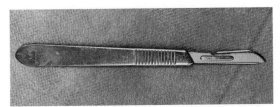

Fig. 2.1 Scalpel; used to cut skin and soft tissue and for sharp dissection.

Annulotomy is typically performed with a No. 15- or 11-blade scalpel followed by removal of disc fragment with pituitary rongeurs (Fig. 2.3), curettes, and Kerrison rongeurs (Fig. 2.4).[2] Several different sized

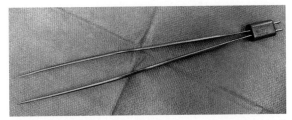

Fig. 2.2 Bipolar cautery; used for coagulation of vasculature and soft tissue for dissection.

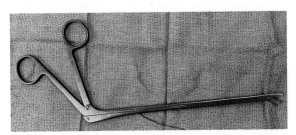

Fig. 2.3 Pituitary rongeur; used to remove soft tissue, disc fragment, bone, or ligamentum flavum for decompression.

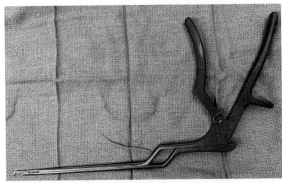

Fig. 2.4 Kerrison rongeur; used to remove soft tissue, disc fragment, bone, or ligamentum flavum for decompression.

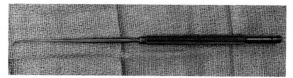

Fig. 2.5 Nerve hook; used to palpate and dissect nerve roots for decompression, as well as blunt microdissection to develop surgical planes with the neural structures during decompression.

cutting and diamond high-speed drill burrs may be used to remove disc fragments and cartilage from the end plates. Ventral decompression of the posterior longitudinal ligament (PLL) may be achieved by establishing a plane from the spinal canal dura with a combination of a nerve hook (Fig. 2.5), curettes, and Kerrison rongeurs.[2]

POSTERIOR APPROACH

Posterior cervical decompression involves removal of posterior bony structures, such as the spinous process, laminae, and superior/inferior articulating processes, in addition to soft tissue structures such as the ligamentum flavum and epidural fat. Several different sized cutting and diamond high-speed drill burrs may be used to remove posterior bony structures, and a combination of a nerve hook, curettes, and Kerrison rongeurs may be used to remove soft tissue that is causing dorsal compression of the cervical spinal cord. There are now trends in MIS surgery toward decompression utilizing muscle-sparing techniques such as tubular decompression with muscle dilatation or utilizing endoscopic techniques to decompress the cervical foramen.

Thoracic Approaches

Thoracic decompressive pathologies may include those of degenerative, congenital, trauma, neoplastic, or infection/inflammatory origin. In the thoracic spine, posterior decompression is achieved via removal of posterior elements, including the spinous process, lamina, and/or decompression of the spinal nerves, called a foraminotomy.[3] Cutting and/or diamond high-speed drill burrs may be used to remove posterior

bony structures, and a combination of a nerve hook, curettes, and Kerrison rongeurs may be used to remove soft tissue that is causing dorsal compression of the thoracic spinal cord. Additionally, to access anterior or lateral compression of the thoracic spinal cord, a costotransversectomy and/or transpedicular approach may be employed by using a high-speed drill and following the superior edge of the pedicle to identify the disc space and decompress from a lateral technique without mobilization of the spinal cord. This can be done using microscopic MIS techniques such as a tubular decompression or other muscle-sparing techniques. The instruments are often similar to traditional open instruments; however, they are "bayoneted" so as not to block the surgeon's view through the working channel. Drills, Woodson elevators, curettes, pituitary rongeurs, and nerve hooks are all available in bayoneted form.

Lumbar/Sacral Approaches

Lumbar decompression may be used to relieve pressure on the spinal cord or canal from compressive bone, ligamentum flavum, facet hypertrophy, epidural fat, disc herniation, malignancy, infection, or other processes. Posterior bony elements are exposed with a Weitlaner retractor (Fig. 2.6), and decompression may be achieved with a high-speed drill or

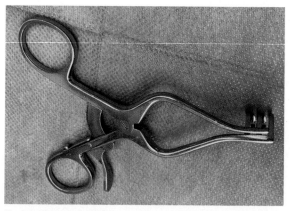

Fig. 2.6 Weitlaner retractor; used for retracting skin and soft tissue to expose the surgical field.

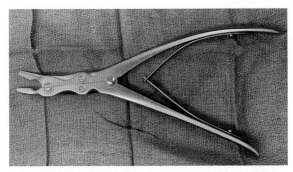

Fig. 2.7 Leksell rongeur; used to remove soft tissue, bone, or ligamentum flavum for decompression.

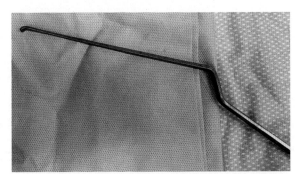

Fig. 2.8 Nerve root retractor; used to retract the spinal canal or nerve root for decompression by removal of disc fragment, bone, or ligamentum flavum.

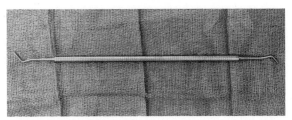

Fig. 2.9 Dental carver instrument; used to palpate and dissect nerve roots for decompression.

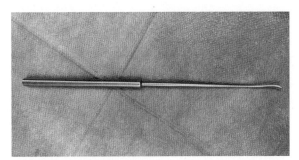

Fig. 2.10 Penfield dissector No. 4; used for microscopic retraction, palpation, and exploration of tissues.

Leksell (Fig. 2.7) and Kerrison rongeurs. Nerve hooks, curettes, and Kerrison rongeurs may be used to remove soft tissue that is causing dorsal compression of the lumbar spinal cord.

When the pathology is due to compression from a disk herniation, an annulotomy is typically performed with a No. 11-blade scalpel followed by removal of disc fragment with pituitary rongeurs, curettes, and Kerrison rongeurs. The thecal sac is retracted gently using a nerve root retractor (Fig. 2.8). To palpate the disc space to ensure there is no more disk or annulus compression of the thecal sac, a dental carver instrument (Fig. 2.9) or Penfield dissector No. 4 (Fig. 2.10) may be used. This can be done in traditional and minimally invasive fashion, similarly to more proximally in the spine.[1]

Closure Techniques

Muscle reapproximation is often performed to promote muscle healing and closure of potential space. Tight fascial closure is important to prevent formation of postoperative seroma collection.[4] Superficial to the fascia, subcuticular layers are often closed with inverted interrupted suture, such as 3-0 Vicryl sutures. In non-CSF leak cases, the skin may be approximated with an absorbable running suture such as Monocryl, with or without the use of skin adhesive. In cases of accidental dural tear, the skin is often approximated with nonabsorbable suture such as Nylon or Prolene to ensure no leakage from the skin and no communication from the intradural space to the skin, which can lead to meningitis.

In the event of CSF leak, when possible, the goal is for primary closure[5]; however, this may not always be feasible. The closure techniques for dural repair are beyond the scope of this chapter.

REFERENCES

1. Bridwell KH. *Textbook of Spinal Surgery*. 4th ed. Philadelphia, PA, USA: Lippincott Williams & Wilkins; 2019.
2. Truumees E, Geck M, Stokes JK, Singh D. Lumbar microdiscectomy. *JBJS Essent Surg Tech*. 2016;6(1):e3.
3. Rane A, Spiker WR, Daubs MD. *Thoracic Decompression and Instrumented Fusion Techniques*. Musculoskeletal Key; 2018. Available at: https://musculoskeletalkey.com/thoracic-decompression-and-instrumented-fusion-techniques/.
4. Yilmaz E, Blecher R, Moisi M, et al. Is there an optimal wound closure technique for major posterior spine surgery? A systematic review. *Global Spine J*. 2018;8(5):535-544.
5. Shenoy K, Donnally CJ III, Sheha ED, Khanna K, Prasad SK. An investigation of a novel dural repair device for intraoperative incidental durotomy repair. *Front Surg*. 2021;8:642972.

Chapter 3

Discectomy: A Surgical Approach

Hamid R. Abbasi, Alaa A. Abd-Elsayed, and Nicholas R. Storlie

Introduction

Lumbar disc herniation (LDH) is the one of the most common diagnoses in spine practice for patients with lower back pain and radiculopathy, with an estimated prevalence of 2%–3%.[1] Disc herniation occurs when the nucleus pulposus is displaced through the annulus fibrosus, which can cause compression and irritation of the nerve roots and spinal cord.[2] Lumbar discectomy, a surgery in which the nervous tissue is directly decompressed through removal of extruded disc, is the most common neurosurgical procedure in the United States.[3] Though historically performed through an open, muscle stripping approach, the procedure has been modified using minimally invasive principles since the introduction of the operating microscope.[4] Microdiscectomy has become the prevalent method of treatment for LDH due to the reduced soft tissue damage from the smaller approach window, while providing comparable patient outcomes.[5,6]

We describe a method of microdiscectomy which accesses the extruded disc utilizing a unilateral approach with a tubular retractor system that provides the surgical window. This approach minimizes iatrogenic muscle splitting while providing adequate visualization of relevant nervous anatomy and tissue. After the tubular retractor has been placed, laminotomy is performed to allow access to the disc. Medial facetectomy and foraminotomy is also oftentimes performed during this procedure to ensure adequate decompression of the nerve root in the foramen and lateral recess.

One divergence in the practice of minimally invasive discectomy is the choice to use a surgical microscope or endoscope for visualization during the procedure. Microscopy is our preferred method because it allows for a three-dimensional view of the operation and the use of both hands during discectomy, whereas endoscopy often needs one hand to stabilize the endoscope.

Indications

Indications of discectomy include:
1. Lower back pain or radiculopathy with evidence of nerve root irritation or neurological deficits.
2. Have undergone and failed intensive nonoperative treatment that includes medication optimization, activity modification, and active physical therapy for treatment of symptoms. In the case of progressive neurological deficit, there is no need for conservative therapy.
3. MRI evidence of moderate to severe central canal and/or lateral recess spinal stenosis related to disc herniation.

Relevant Contraindications

Microdiscectomy can be contraindicated in any of the following scenarios:
1. Presence of unstable spinal anatomy due to spondylolisthesis, lateral listhesis, or scoliosis.
2. Presence of concurrent pathology such as tumor or infection.
3. Revision cases with extensive surgical scarring, which increases the risk of surgery dramatically.

Preoperative Considerations

Preoperatively, the patient is induced and placed in the prone position on a Jackson table. The area around the patient's targeted surgical level is prepared and the draping is performed prior to surgery. Intraoperatively, 1% lidocaine with epinephrine and 0.25% Marcaine plain mixed 1:1 is injected at the skin where the incision will be made.

Postoperative Care

The surgery can be performed in an outpatient setting, and the patient is usually discharged the same day. The patient is discharged with pain medication and muscle relaxants.

Complications

Complications of microdiscectomy include:
1. Violation of the thecal sac and nerve roots can result in iatrogenic damage to nerves and cerebrospinal fluid leak.
   a. This risk can be minimized by ensuring there is no adhesion of the dura to the ligamentum flavum and **removing the ligamentum flavum after contralateral decompression.**
   b. Durotomy should be repaired if possible, directly with 4-0 Nurolon sutures. Hydrogel dural sealant (DuraSeal) may be sufficient to close the dura in smaller cases.
2. Postoperative hematoma manifesting as progressively worsening neurological symptoms.
   a. Emergent MRI should be performed to rule out hematoma, and emergency decompression may be necessary.
3. Infection of the surgical site requiring antibiotics.

Microdiscectomy

EQUIPMENT

Equipment needed are summarized in Figs. 3.1–3.4.

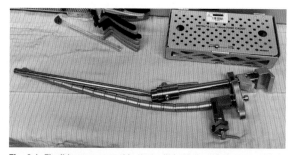

Fig. 3.1 Flexible arm assembly that will hold the tubular retractor in place during the surgery.

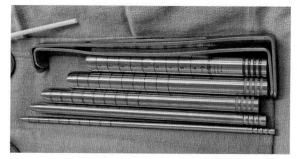

Fig. 3.2 Sequential dilators and retractors.

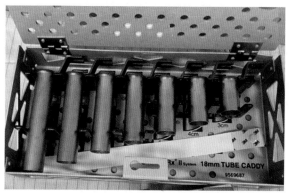

Fig. 3.3 Various depths of tubular retractors.

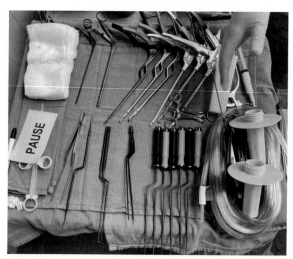

Fig. 3.4 Curettes, Kerrisons, and other instruments used during surgery.

ANATOMY (FIG. 3.5)

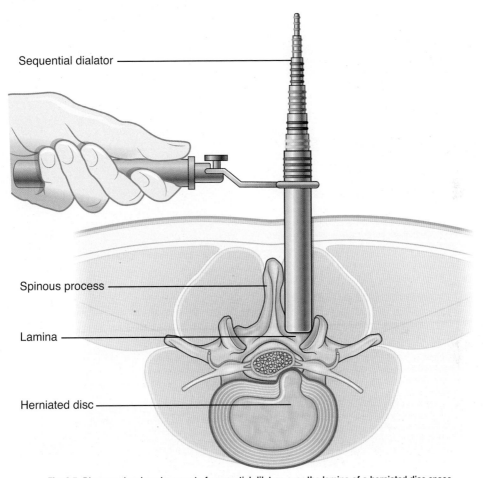

Sequential dialator

Spinous process

Lamina

Herniated disc

Fig. 3.5 Diagram showing placement of sequential dilators over the lamina of a herniated disc space.

SETUP (FIGS. 3.6, 3.7)

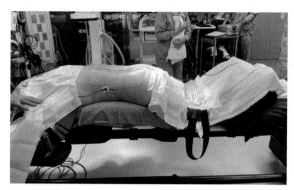

Fig. 3.6 Patient is placed in the prone position on a Jackson table. The patient is draped and the targeted area is sterilized. The surgeon will stand on the side of the patient where the herniation will be treated.

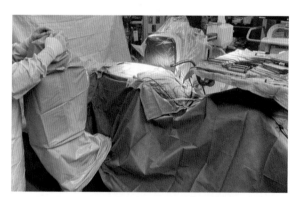

Fig. 3.7 Lateral X-ray is used in this procedure.

ACCESSING THE DISC (FIGS. 3.8–3.22)

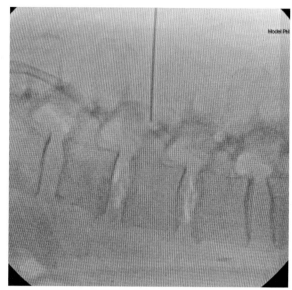

Fig. 3.8 Spinal needle is placed to identify the targeted level.

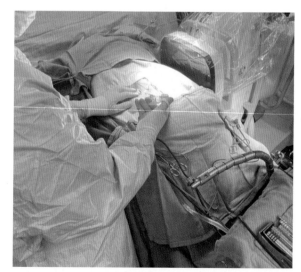

Fig. 3.9 Mixture of 0.25% Marcaine and epinephrine is injected into the skin over the targeted disc. A small 0.5–1 inch incision should be made to allow for the desired dilator to fit.

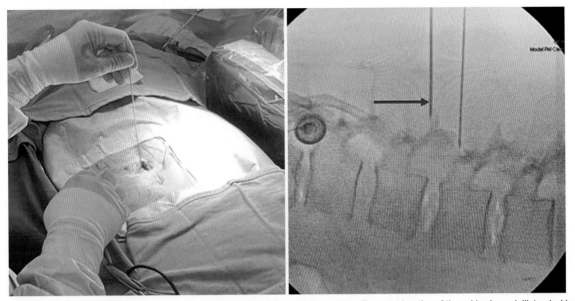

Fig. 3.10 Guidewire is advanced to the inferior edge of the lamina of the superior vertebra. The exact location of the guidewire and dilator docking point is determined by the location of the disc herniation as determined by MRI.

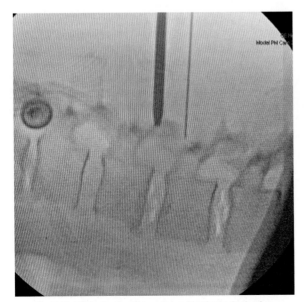

Fig. 3.11 Dilator is placed over the guidewire to the lamina.

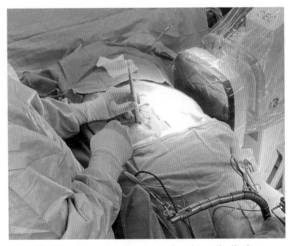

Fig. 3.12 Sequential dilators are placed over the K-wire.

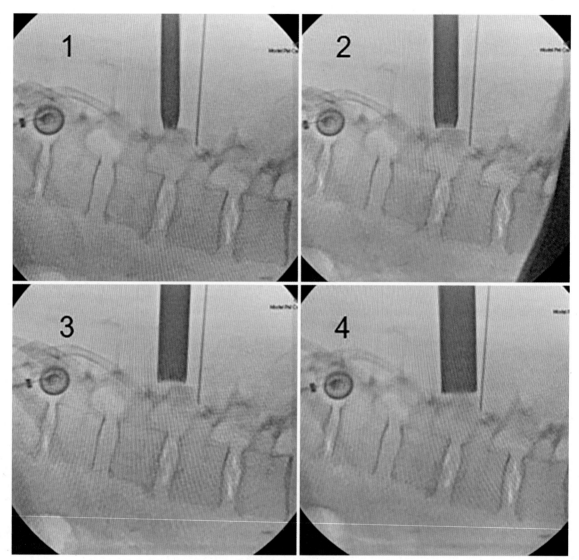

Fig. 3.13 Lateral X-ray of sequential dilation being placed to access the disc space.

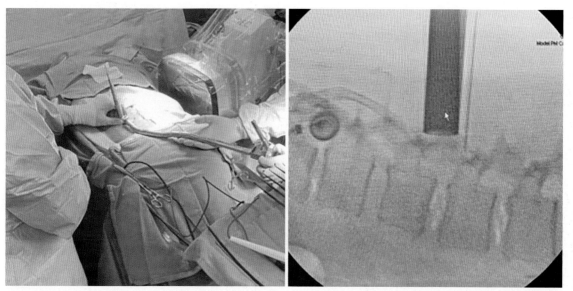

Fig. 3.14 An 18-mm tubular retractor, connected to the flexible arm, is placed over the sequential dilators down to the target disc space.

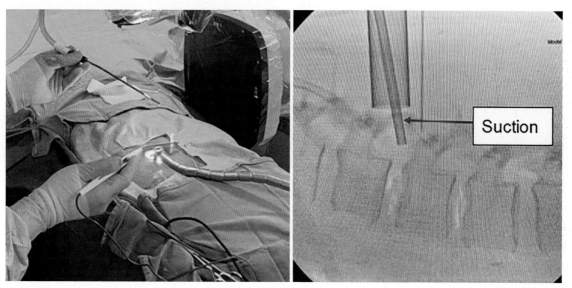

Fig. 3.15 Dilators are removed, and the tubular retractor (held in place by the flexible arm) is used as an operative window to the disc space. Correct placement of the tubular retractor is confirmed with fluoroscopy.

After the tubular retractor is placed, high-speed drill and Kerrison rongeur are used to perform a laminotomy and visualize the ligamentum flavum.

Medial facetectomy is also performed to better visualize the dura and nerve root and provide decompression.

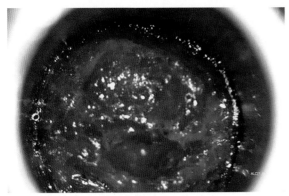

Fig. 3.16 Microscope view through the tubular retractor to the paraspinal muscles covering the facet joint.

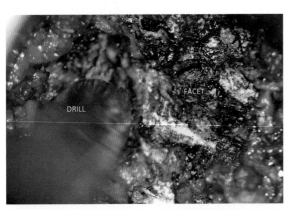

Fig. 3.17 Microscope image of drill being used to perform medial facetectomy.

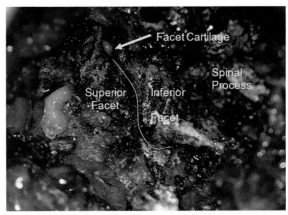

Fig. 3.18 Microscope image with the facet partially removed.

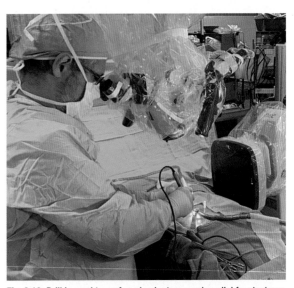

Fig. 3.19 Drill is used to perform laminotomy and medial facetectomy.

Part of the ligamentum flavum is dissected with a ball-tipped dissector and then removed with a Kerrison rongeur to visualize the dura. After the nerve root has been visualized, and retracted if necessary, it is possible to dissect to the disc and begin discectomy. Bipolar cautery can be used at a low setting (10–15 mA) for hemostasis and to shrink fat.

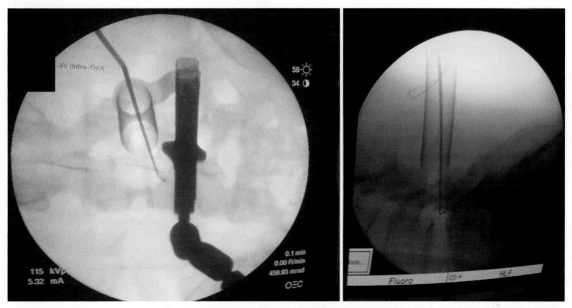

Fig. 3.20 Ligamentum flavum is dissected prior to resection.

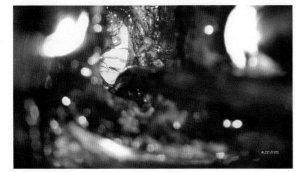

Fig. 3.21 Ligamentum flavum being removed from the dura.

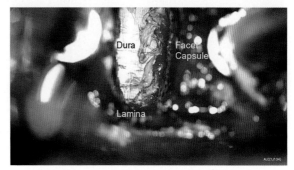

Fig. 3.22 The dura is visualized after medial facetectomy.

DISCECTOMY

After the disc mass has been exposed, pieces of disc are removed with right-angled curettes and various sizes of pituitary rongeurs. A bayoneted scalpel is used to incise the annulus if necessary. It is important not to violate the anterior annulus to avoid vascular injury (Fig. 3.23).

CLOSING (FIG. 3.24)

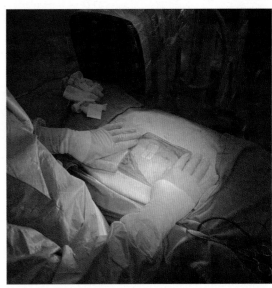

Fig. 3.24 Patient is sutured and bandaged following microdiscectomy.

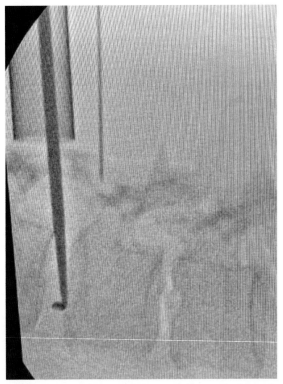

Fig. 3.23 Lateral X-ray of curette being used to remove disc fragments.

REFERENCES

1. Vialle LR, Vialle EN, Henao JE, Giraldo G. Lumbar disc herniation. *Rev Bras Ortop*. 2010;45(1):17-22.
2. Amin RM, Andrade NS, Neuman BJ. Lumbar disc herniation. *Curr Rev Musculoskelet Med*. 2017;10(4):507-516.
3. Koebbe CJ, Maroon JC, Abla A, El-Kadi H, Bost J. Lumbar microdiscectomy: a historical perspective and current technical considerations. *Neurosurg Focus*. 2002;13(2):1-6.
4. Rasouli MR, Rahimi-Movaghar V, Shokraneh F, Moradi-Lakeh M, Chou R. Minimally invasive discectomy versus microdiscectomy/open discectomy for symptomatic lumbar disc herniation. *Cochrane Database Syst Rev*. 2014;(9):CD010328.
5. Veresciagina K, Spakauskas B, Ambrozaitis KV. Clinical outcomes of patients with lumbar disc herniation, selected for one-level open-discectomy and microdiscectomy. *Eur Spine J*. 2010;19(9):1450-1458.
6. Clark AJ, Safaee MM, Khan NR, Brown MT, Foley KT. Tubular microdiscectomy: techniques, complication avoidance, and review of the literature. *Neurosurg Focus*. 2017;43(2):1-9.

Chapter 4

Methods for Percutaneous Discectomy

Christopher Robinson, Nasir Hussain, and Alaa A. Abd-Elsayed

Introduction

Acute back pain can be severe and debilitating, and if not appropriately treated, can lead to recurrent symptoms in the majority of paitents.[1] One of the leading causes of back pain is intervertebral degeneration that can lead to degenerative disease and disc herniation.[2] Disc herniation results from a localized displacement of the nucleus pulposus beyond the margins of the intervertebral disc space.[3] Treatments for disc herniations include conservative medical management and physical therapy. More interventional approaches can also be considered, including epidural or transforaminal steroid injections[3]; however, when symptoms are resistant to these measures, more invasive interventions including discectomy and surgery can be considered to remove the herniated disc.[4,5]

Although there is controversy over the superiority of surgical intervention versus conservative management, roughly 40% of patients receiving conservative management will eventually undergo a surgical intervention to treat the herniated disc.[6,7] When surgical intervention occurs, nearly 18% of patients will experience a recurrence of the disc herniation, which is defined as a pain-free period of minimum of 6 months with herniation at the same level, and 80% of these patients will undergo a second operation.[8-13] Though neither discectomy nor surgical management has been found to be superior, the question to continue conservative measures and tolerate the symptoms, or proceed with discectomy or surgical intervention remains a predicament to both the patient and the physician.[3] If discectomy is determined to be the treatment method, several different techniques can be considered.[13] In this chapter, we will explore the indications, clinical applications, technical approaches, and complications for minimally invasive discectomy techniques for the treatment of disc herniations.

Relevant Anatomy

The intervertebral disc is composed of an outer annulus fibrosus with an inner nucleus pulposus that is the site of collagen secretion; it consists mainly of type II collagen, which accounts for 20% of its dry weight (Fig. 4.1).[14] The nucleus pulposus contains proteoglycans that retain water to provide cushioning to resist axial compression of the spine.[15,16] The purpose of the annulus fibrosus, which is composed mainly of type I collagen, is to maintain the central location of the nucleus pulposus.[15,17,18] The spinal canal or foraminal space can be become narrowed when (1) there is disc protrusion causing possible impingement of the thecal sac or exiting spinal nerve roots when an entire disc protrudes with an intact annulus fibrosus; (2) the

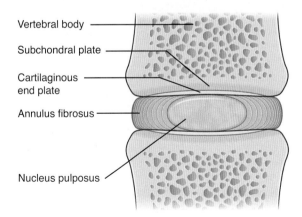

Vertebral body

Subchondral plate

Cartilaginous end plate

Annulus fibrosus

Nucleus pulposus

Fig. 4.1 The anatomy of the intervertebral disc with the nucleus pulposus in the center surrounded by the annulus fibrosus between the vertebral bones.

nucleus pulposus protrudes through a disrupted annulus fibrosus; or (3) the nucleus pulposus protrudes and breaks off as a free segment (Fig. 4.2).[14]

Biological factors that increase the risk of disc herniation include reduction of water in the nucleus pulposus, increase in the amount of type I collagen in both the nucleus pulposus and annulus fibrosus, degradation of collagen and extracellular matrix, and an upregulation of matrix metalloproteinase and inflammatory pathways.[14,17,19-22] Up to 75% of individuals affected by disc herniation are estimated to be predisposed to the condition as numerous genes are

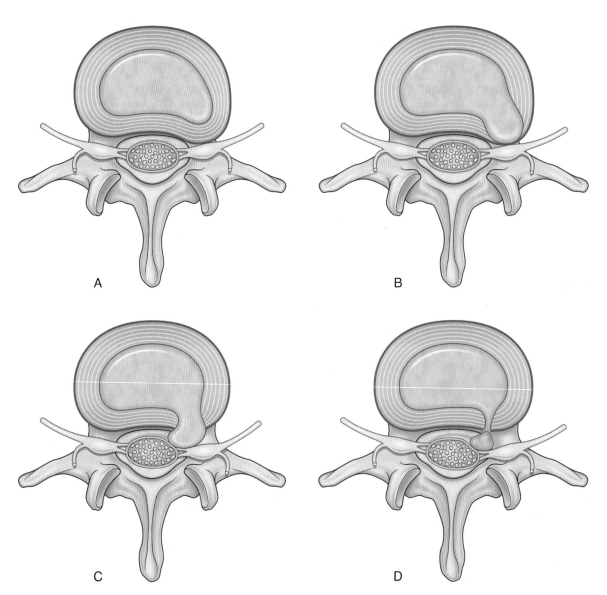

Fig. 4.2 The different types of disc herniations. (A) contained disc herniation, (B) lateral herniation impingement on the nerve root, (C) lateral herniation with disrupted annulus fibrosus, and (D) central herniation impinging on the spinal cord.

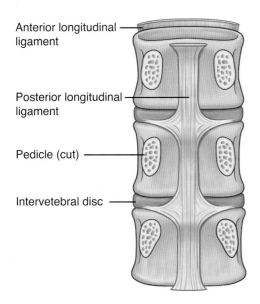

Anterior longitudinal
ligament

Posterior longitudinal
ligament

Pedicle (cut)

Intervetebral disc

Fig. 4.3 The location of the posterior and anterior longitudinal ligaments. The posterior longitudinal ligament is a single layer, thinner, and less developed laterally as compared with the anterior longitudinal ligament.

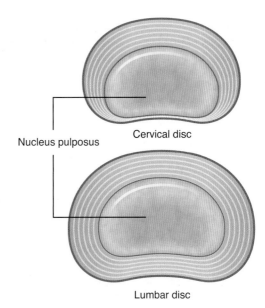

Nucleus pulposus

Cervical disc

Lumbar disc

Fig. 4.4 The location of the nucleus pulposus in the cervical and thoracic spine. The lumbar nucleus pulposus sits more posteriorly than the cervical nucleus pulposus.

involved in weakening and changing the structures involved in disc herniations.[23] Aside from biologic and genetic factors, disc herniations can result from axial overloading without any predisposing factors or degeneration.[24] Without predisposing factors, the herniation of discs can occur from spinal overloading, especially from static overloading, which increases risk for posterior disc herniation.[25-27] The static overloading may be the culprit in the increasing prevalence of disc herniation in sedentary, younger individuals who spend most of their time in the seated position.[26]

The most common area for disc herniations is the lumbar spine followed by the cervical spine with the thoracic region having the lowest incidence of disc herniation.[28-30] The discs are more likely to herniate posterolaterally where the annulus fibrosus is thinner and lacks the support from posterior longitudinal ligament (Figs. 4.2, 4.3).[28] Additionally, lumbar roots are not protected from impingement from herniation by the bony wall of the facet joints as cervical joints are, and the nuclear material is more posterior than its cervical counterparts (Fig. 4.4).[31]

Clinical Presentation and Diagnosis

The symptoms of disc herniation include radicular pain, sensory abnormalities in a dermatomal distribution, weakness in the distribution of one or more nerve roots, focal paresis, limited flexion, and pain associated with increased intraabdominal/thoracic pressure.[32,33] When the herniation is paracentral, the traversing nerves roots are affected. In contrast, when it is a far lateral herniation, the exiting nerve root can be affected.[14]

Diagnostic criteria for lumbar disc herniation was recommended by the Lumbar Disc Herniation with Radiculopathy Work Group of the North American Spine Society's (NASS) Evidence-Based Guideline Development Committee to consist of manual muscle testing, sensory testing, and supine leg raise test as the gold standard for diagnosis.[34] Other recommendations include screening with the straight leg test, and if three of the four symptoms are present (dermatomal pain, sensory deficits, reflex deficits, and motor weakness), then a diagnosis of lumbar disc herniation can be made.[35] Plain radiographs are also commonly performed as a first-line imaging modality for back pain with findings such as narrowed intervertebral space, presence of traction osteophytes, and compensatory scoliosis indicative of disc herniation.[14] MRI, however, is the gold standard to confirm a disc herniation with an accuracy of 97%.[34,36] Findings include enhanced T2-weighted signal from the posterior 10% of the disc diameter.[37]

Conservative Treatment

Conservative medical management of disc herniations is often multimodal and includes antiinflammatory medications and physical therapy, with hopeful resolution weeks after the onset of symptoms.[38] Though often prescribed, limited evidence exists for the use of muscle relaxants and oral corticosteroids.[39] When symptoms last for >6 weeks, translaminar epidural steroid injections, a second-line treatment, can be considered. Though reductions in pain and function can be immediate, often the benefits are limited in duration, and patients require repeated injections with minimal effect on the long-term risk of surgery.[40,41] Epidural steroid injection can also be considered, but the long-term benefits may be limited.[42] Even if these methods improve symptoms, the risk of disc reherniation is elevated and is increased by the following risk factors: diabetes, advanced age, smoking, trauma, preoperative disc height index, disc sequestration, longer duration of sick leave, workers' compensation, and greater preoperative symptom severity.[43-49]

Minimally Invasive Treatment

If conservative and epidural injections fail, operative management can be considered; although this has short-term benefits, benefits in the long term are conflicting.[7,50,51] Interestingly, various factors can predict successful outcomes after discectomy, and include severe acute preoperative low back pain, increased preoperative physical activity, younger age, shorter symptom duration, mental health status, and higher preoperative leg pain severity.[14,43,52,53] An invasive surgical method, the open discectomy, has demonstrated efficacy in treating lumbar disc herniations.[7,50] Based on the herniation location (paracentral or far

lateral), different approaches can be considered. The paracentral approach results in longer incisions, more muscle stripping, and is limited due to the difficulty in accessing far lateral discectomy.[54] For far lateral, the Wiltse paraspinal approach can be performed.[55] As with all forms of surgical intervention, minimally invasive techniques for discectomy have been increasingly utilized over the past years.

Minimally invasive techniques used by interventional chronic pain specialists have been found to be associated with a reduction in length of hospital stay, less trauma to the tissue and bones, and lower acute care charges.[56] When compared to open discectomy, these minimally invasive techniques result in a decreased operative time, less blood loss, fewer complications, lower reoperation rates, and fewer infections.[57] Minimally invasive techniques include percutaneous discectomy automated technique and laser-assisted technique, percutaneous laser-assisted annuloplasty, minimally invasive lumbar decompression procedure, and percutaneous endoscopic lumbar discectomy performed via the transforaminal or interlaminar approach. The following sections will summarize each approach with associated complications.

Percutaneous Discectomy: Automated Technique[58]

Percutaneous discectomy using the automated technique is indicated for patients with low back and radicular pain caused by a contained disc protrusion who have failed medical management (Figs. 4.5, 4.6).[59] To perform the technique, the patient is positioned in the lateral or prone position with slight flexion of the lumbar spine, which can be assisted by placing a pillow under the abdomen. The spinous processes of the vertebra to be targeted are identified under fluoroscopic view. The skin is cleaned antiseptically and anesthetized below and laterally 3.8 cm from the spinous processes. A small stab wound is made to allow for the introducer cannula. Under fluoroscopic guidance and sequential imaging, the cannula with the stylet is advanced to the middle of the disc to be decompressed (Figs. 4.6, 4.7). Since the somatic nerve roots are in close proximity, if any paresthesias are elicited, the introducer should be redirected more cephalad. Special care must be taken to

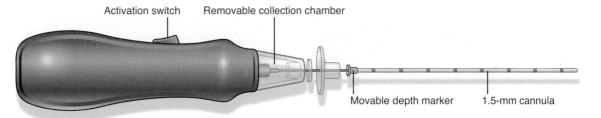

Activation switch   Removable collection chamber

Movable depth marker   1.5-mm cannula

Fig. 4.5 Schematic of the automated decompressor probe used in the percutaneous discectomy automated technique.

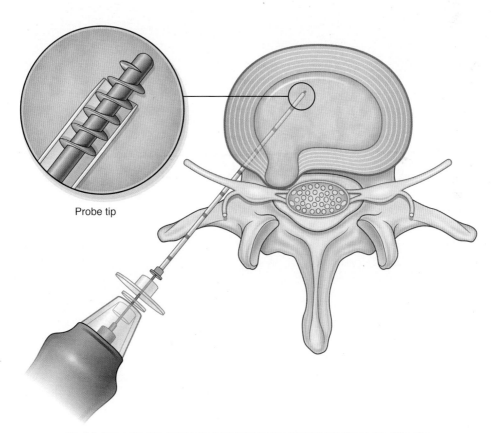

Probe tip

Fig. 4.6 Schematic showing the decompressor probe advancing into the center of the disc.

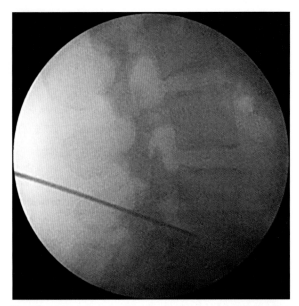

Fig. 4.7 A lateral fluoroscopic image showing the cannula in the disc. (From Waldman SD. *Atlas of Interventional Pain Management*. 5th ed. Philadelphia, PA: Elsevier; 2020: p. 1033.)

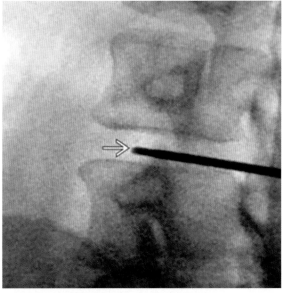

Fig. 4.8 A lateral fluoroscopic image with the cannula in the center of the disc immediately before contrast is injected to confirm its location. (From Ross JS. Percutaneous discectomy. In: Ross JS, Bendok BR, McClendon J Jr, eds. Imaging in Spine Surgery. Philadelphia: Elsevier; 2017:468–469.)

not advance the needle completely through the disc or into the lower limits of the spinal cord or cauda equina. If advanced too laterally, the needle can enter the lower pleura or retroperitoneum. With the cannula in the center of the disc, the stylet is then removed, and contrast is injected to assess for any annulus abnormalities (Fig. 4.8). The decompressor probe is then advanced until it exits the cannula. The probe is activated for 15 seconds at a time for a maximum total of 5 minutes. The probe can then be slowly advanced to the anterior annulus without impinging on it. After sufficient disc has been removed, the probe can be withdrawn.

ASSOCIATED COMPLICATIONS

Complications tend to be self-limited. Discitis, which can be difficult to treat due to the limited blood supply to the disc, can occur, and presents with spine pain days to weeks after the procedure. Epidural abscess can occur 24–48 hours after the procedure and presents with fever, severe back pain, and neurological deficits. Both complications require further investigation with urine and blood samples, initiation of

empiric antibiotics, and emergent MRI for possible drainage. Rarely, pneumothorax can occur, but it is typically limited with the use of fluoroscopic techniques. If small in size, pneumothorax can be treated conservatively, but if significant, it may require placement of a chest tube. Retroperitoneal organ damage can occur but is minimized with fluoroscopic visualization during the procedure. Finally, spinal cord damage can occur if the needle goes through the entire disc, and nerve root damage can occur if the needle is advanced too laterally.

Percutaneous Discectomy: Laser-Assisted Technique[31]

Percutaneous discectomy using the laser-assisted technique is indicated in patients with low back and radicular pain caused by disc protrusion. This technique vaporizes portions of the herniated disc with energy derived from the laser in an attempt to reduce intradiscal pressure (Fig. 4.9). Like percutaneous discectomy using the automated technique, patients must have failed conservative management and epidural

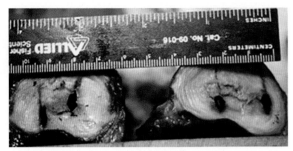

Fig. 4.9 A gross specimen of the discs demonstrating laser tracts. (From Choy DSJ, Tassi GP, Hellinger J, et al. Twenty-three years of percutaneous laser disc decompression (PLDD)—state of the art and future prospects. Med Laser Appl. 2009;24[3]:147–157.)

steroids with some chronic pain specialists recommending a trial of transforaminal epidural steroid injection. However, unlike percutaneous discectomy using the automated technique, computed tomography (CT) is preferred over fluoroscopic guidance, as CT can demonstrate the vaporization of the nuclear material. Positioning is similar to the automated technique. Several CT images are first taken near the disc to be treated to assess the positions of the surrounding structures. The skin over the lumbar paraspinous regions is prepared antiseptically and anesthetized. The introducer is then inserted and directed under CT guidance toward the annulus and posterior disc to be treated, with needle placement confirmed by CT (Fig. 4.10). Once in the proper place, the fiberoptic cable is placed through the introducer and advanced until it exits and extends beyond the introducer by approximately 5–6 mm. The settings for the vaporizer are 15–20 W delivered in 0.5–1.0 second pulses at four 10-second intervals with a total dose of 1200–1500 J.

ASSOCIATED COMPLICATIONS

Complications are similar to percutaneous discectomy using the automated technique and include discitis, epidural abscess, pneumothorax, and spinal cord and nerve root injury. Osteonecrosis has been reported of the adjacent vertebral body and is more often seen when a side-firing potassium triphosphide or holmium:yttrium-aluminum-garnet laser is used. It is less frequent when a direct-firing neodymium-doped yttrium-aluminum-garnet laser is used.

Percutaneous Laser-Assisted Annuloplasty[60]

Percutaneous laser-assisted annuloplasty is indicated in patients with lumbar discogenic pain secondary to an internally disrupted disc or limited herniation that

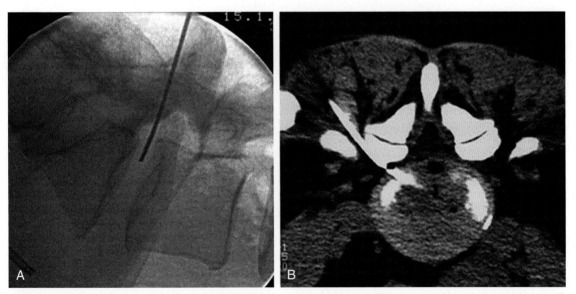

Fig. 4.10 Lateral fluoroscopic image (A) of the needle positioned in the nucleus pulposus. (B) CT image taken during the vaporization step. (From Waldman SD. *Atlas of Interventional Pain Management.* 5th ed. Philadelphia, PA: Elsevier; 2020: p. 1042.)

fails to respond to medical management and epidural steroid injections. It is believed to cause pain relief via destruction of annular nociceptive fibers, thermal injury to the annulus with healing afterwards, and reduction of disc volume and pressure. It is not indicated in patients with spinal stenosis or disc herniation with nerve root impingement.

The patient can be positioned in the prone or lateral position based on the choice of the chronic pain specialist. If prone positioning is chosen, then the patient can be placed in a partially oblique position with a foam wedge. The skin is then prepared and anesthetized, and the inferior end plate of the affected spinal level is located under fluoroscope guidance. The fluoroscope beam is rotated to locate the superior articular process, and the beam is aligned to the middle-inferior aspect of the end plate. The needle should enter the skin lateral to the middle of the superior articular process and advanced anterior to the midpoint of the superior articular surface and parallel to the endplates. Additional anesthetic can be injected at this time to assist with procedural discomfort. The introducer is inserted parallel to the needle, advanced into the posterior annulus, and the tip location confirmed by taking fluoroscopic images in multiple planes.

Discography should then be performed to locate the exact area to be treated and determine annular abnormalities. This can be done with 0.3 mL of contrast mixed with 0.3 mL of sterile indigo carmine, which will highlight the diseased annular ring (Fig. 4.11). Finally, after endoscopic assessment and under fluoroscopy, the fiberoptic cable is then introduced into the subligamentous portion of the posterior annulus (Fig. 4.12). The settings for the holmium:yttrium-aluminum-garnet laser should be set between 0.5 and 1.2 J to provide up to 11,000 J. Depending on the experience and preference of the chronic pain specialist, intradiscal

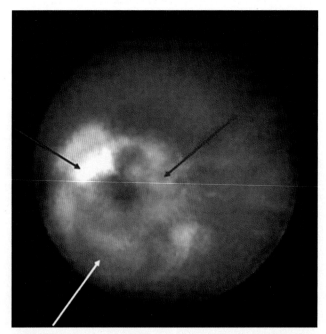

Fig. 4.11 Endoscopic image taken after injection of contrast and indigo carmine that stains the granulation tissue. *Blue arrow* indicates the injected dye, *white arrow* demonstrates the healthy annulus, and *red arrow* is the laser tip. (From Lee SH, Kang HS. Percutaneous endoscopic laser annuloplasty for discogenic low back pain. World Neurosurg. 2010;73[3]:198–206.)

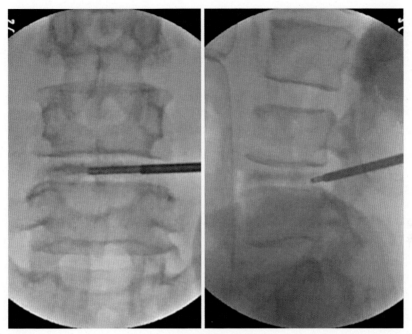

Fig. 4.12 Fluoroscopic images confirming the proper location of the needle and catheter intraannularly. *Left,* Anterioposterior view; *Right,* lateral view. (From Lee SH, Kang HS. Percutaneous endoscopic laser annuloplasty for discogenic low back pain. World Neurosurg. 2010;73[3]:198–206.)

antibiotics and/or steroids can be injected prior to full removal of the introducer.

ASSOCIATED COMPLICATIONS

Of note, back or radicular pain can worsen following the procedure and last for 3–7 days. Treatment involves reassurance and if needed, typical analgesics. Relief of postprocedural pain should occur gradually over 4–6 weeks. After 2–3 months, physical therapy should be recommended. Other complications are similar to the aforementioned procedures; thermal injury to nearby structures may also occur.

Percutaneous Intradiscal Nucleoplasty[61]

Percutaneous intradiscal nucleoplasty is indicated in patients who have low back and radicular pain due to a contained disc protrusion and have failed conservative management and epidural steroid injections (Fig. 4.13). Some chronic pain specialists recommend a trial of transforaminal epidural steroid injections prior to proceeding with this route. Negative predictors of

success include obesity and discogenic disease at multiple levels.

Percutaneous intradiscal nucleoplasty can be performed under fluoroscopy or CT guidance. CT offers the benefit of better identification of anatomic structures and positions. The patient is positioned similarly to the other techniques, with flexion of the lumbar spine. The skin is prepared antiseptically at a point below and 3.8 cm lateral to the spinous process. Prior to insertion, the stylet is removed from a 17-gauge, 6-inch styletted Crawford needle, and a cryoablation wand is placed into the needle until its reference mark is positioned at the proximal edge of the needle hub, indicating the maximal distance for creating coablation channels. The stylet is then reinserted into the Crawford needle, and the needle is inserted into the skin and advanced toward the middle of the disc until the tip rests against or slightly through the annulus of the affected disc (Fig. 4.14). Like the other percutaneous discectomy procedures, care must be taken to avoid injuring the spinal cord, nerve roots, or retroperitoneal structures. The stylet is then removed and the coablation wand

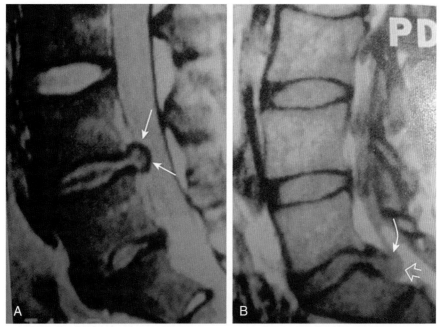

Fig. 4.13 MRI image (A) two white arrows pointing at herniated disc contained within the annulus fibrosus versus (B) solid arrow showing the annulus fibrosus. Hollow arrow showing the herniated disc not contained with the annulus fibrosus. (From Waldman SD. *Atlas of Interventional Pain Management*. 5th ed. Philadelphia, PA: Elsevier; 2020: p. 1015.)

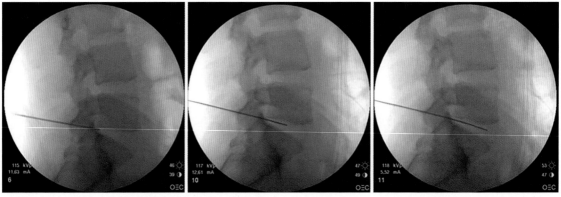

Fig. 4.14 Sequential fluoroscopic images as the needle is advanced into the disc of interest. (From Vivian DG. Intradiscal and peridiscal therapies for discogenic and radicular pain. In: Lennard TA, Walkowski SA, Singla AK, Vivian D, eds. Pain Procedures in Clinical Practice. 3rd ed. Philadelphia: Saunders; 2011:461–482.)

is advanced until the reference mark is at the needle hub. It then is advanced further until it encounters the interior wall of the anterior annulus, as confirmed with fluoroscopy. The wand is then withdrawn and confirmed with fluoroscopy to lie within the disc nucleus. While under the ablation mode, the wand is oriented to the 12 o'clock position. It is then advanced and stopped until it reaches the distal limit and is withdrawn again. Several other channels can be created at the 4, 6, 8, and 10 o'clock positions (Fig. 4.15). Once completed, a post-percutaneous intradiscal nucleoplasty discogram can be performed to evaluate the channels created, or if CT is used, the channels can be visualized directly (Figs. 4.16–4.19).

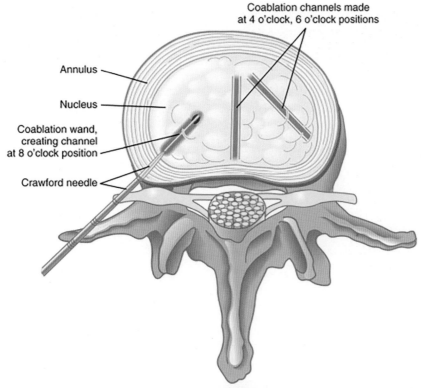

Coablation channels made
at 4 o'clock, 6 o'clock positions

Annulus

Nucleus

Coablation wand,
creating channel
at 8 o'clock position

Crawford needle

Fig. 4.15 Illustration showing the positions in which coablation channels are made. (From Waldman SD. *Atlas of Interventional Pain Management.* 5th ed. Philadelphia, PA: Elsevier; 2020: p. 1020.)

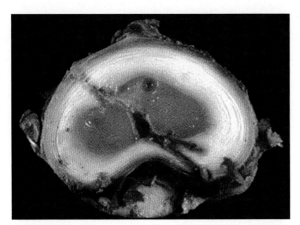

Fig. 4.16 Cross section of lumbar disc showing the channels created during percutaneous intradiscal nucleoplasty. (From Chen YC, Lee SH, Saenz Y, Lehman NL. Histologic findings of disc, end plate and neural elements after coablation of nucleus pulposus: an experimental nucleoplasty study. Spine J. 2003;3[6]:466–470.)

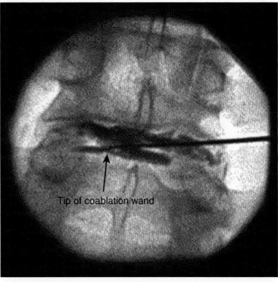

Tip of coablation wand

Fig. 4.17 Discogram performed after an ablation channel is created. (From Kim PS. Nucleoplasty. Tech Reg Anesth Pain Manage. 2004;8[1]: 46–52)

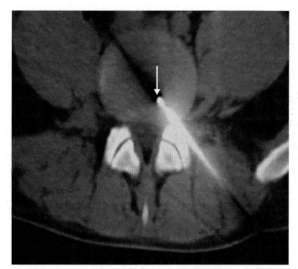

Fig. 4.18 CT showing the advancement of the coablation wand until the tip impinges on the interior wall of the anterior disc annulus. (From Andreula C, Muto M, Leonardi M. Interventional spinal procedures. Eur J Radiol 2004;50[2]:112–119.)

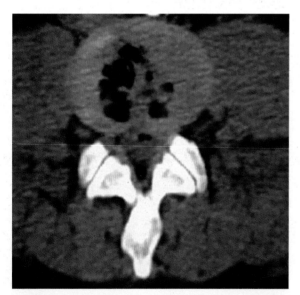

Fig. 4.19 CT showing the ablation channels that are created in the treated disc. (From Andreula C, Muto M, Leonardi M. Interventional spinal procedures. Eur J Radiol 2004;50[2]:112–119.)

ASSOCIATED COMPLICATIONS

Complications are similar to the other procedures and include discitis, epidural abscess, pneumothorax, spinal cord, and nerve root damage.

Percutaneous Endoscopic Lumbar Discectomy[62,63]

TRANSFORAMINAL APPROACH

The transforaminal approach is indicated in patients with lateral-type disc herniations and prior revision surgery. The approach is performed under local anesthesia with 0.5% lidocaine injections, and if necessary, monitored anesthesia care can be performed. The patient is placed in the prone position with genuflex and hip-flexion. Under fluoroscopy, the exact locations for needle insertion are determined. A horizontal line is drawn parallel to the interlaminar space, and a vertical line is made along the ventral edge of the articular process. The boundaries of these two lines are considered the safe area for needle puncture. The needle is then inserted 12–15 cm from the midline, generally superior to the iliac crest at an angle 15–25 degrees to the skin (Fig. 4.20).[64] Occasionally, the crista iliaca can block the path of the needle; if this occurs, the entry angle can be increased, and the insertion point can be more medial. The target of the needle is the medial pedicular line when view in the anterioposterior view and the posterior vertebral line when viewed laterally.

An epidurography is then performed to visualize the location of the exiting and transversing root. The needle is advanced toward the extruded disc, and 0.5% lidocaine is injected. The needle is then advanced further to the center of the disc. Once in place, the needle stylet is removed, and a mixture of contrast and methylthioninium chloride (3:1) is injected for discography. A guidewire is inserted through the needle, and the needle is then removed. Next, a 0.7-cm incision is made at the insertion of the needle at the skin, and a dilator and cannula are inserted through the guidewire. If leg pain occurs during insertion, the angle is adjusted to avoid nerve root damage. If the cannula is blocked by the facet joint, the intervertebral foramen can be enlarged by the usage of trephine. As the cannula reaches the annulus, it is inserted into the disc. Once the cannula

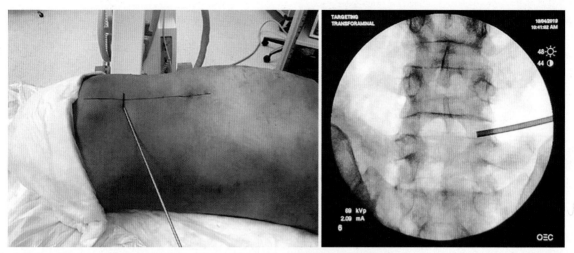

Fig. 4.20 An initial angle of 15–20 degrees is used to insert the needle *(left)* and is confirmed under fluoroscopy *(right)* when performing the per-cutaneous endoscopic transforaminal discectomy. (Image courtesy Elliquence. https://www.elliquence.com/)

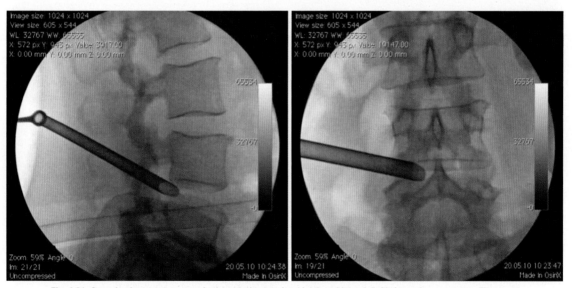

Fig. 4.21 Cannula placement as seen in the anteriposterior *(right)* and lateral *(left)* views. (Image courtesy Elliquence.)

is properly inserted and confirmed (Fig. 4.21), the endoscope can be placed through the cannula, and Ellman electrodes can be used to remove residual fascia and ligaments. The previously stained degenerative pulposus is removed (Fig. 4.22), and the decompressed nerve root is visualized (Fig. 4.23).

Topical glucocorticoids are applied to reduce any nerve root inflammation. Due to possible blockade by the crista iliaca and narrow foramen, the transforaminal approach can lead to longer operative times and as a result, more radiation exposure with the possibility of failure of the procedure.[65,66]

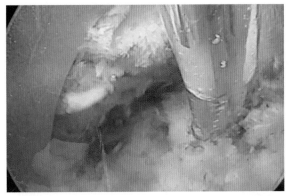

Fig. 4.22 Endoscopic view of the disc removal during the percutaneous endoscopic transforaminal discectomy. (Image courtesy Elliquence.)

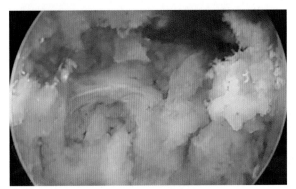

Fig. 4.23 Endoscopic view of the decompressed nerve root after percutaneous endoscopic transforaminal discectomy. (Image courtesy Elliquence.)

INTERLAMINAR APPROACH

The interlaminar approach is indicated in patients with a sequestered disc herniation at the L5–S1 level and is performed under general anesthesia (Fig. 4.24). The patient is placed in the prone position with genuflex and hip-flexion to open up the interlaminar space. The lumbar process is located under fluoroscopy to designate the posterior midline. A needle is then inserted 1 cm lateral to the posterior midline and advanced until the medial side of the facet joint is reached. A 0.8-cm incision is made at the insertion point of the needle at the skin, and a dilator is inserted. A cannula is then placed over the dilator, and the location is confirmed via fluoroscopy at the anteriorposterior and lateral projections. Once confirmed,

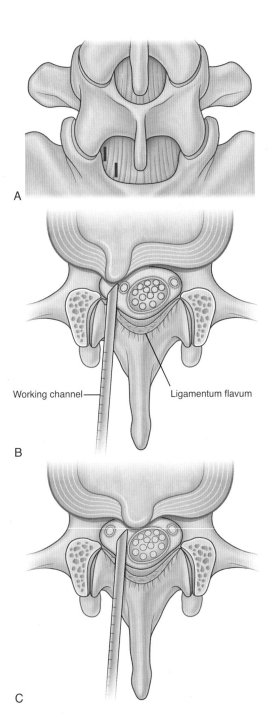

Working channel—   —Ligamentum flavum

Fig. 4.24 Illustration demonstrating the interlaminar approach to microdisectomy. (A) Location of insertion (two red lines) of the working channel into the ligamentum flavum. (B) Showing the technique with a paracentral disc herniation and (C) with a central disc herniation.

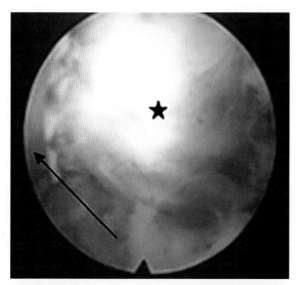

Fig. 4.25 Endoscopic view in the interlaminar approach of the nerve root *(star)* prior to it being pushed away by the working sheath *(long arrow)*. (From Hsu HT, Yang SS. Full-endoscopic interlaminar discectomy for herniation at L3–4 and L4–5: technical note. *Formosan J of Surg.* 2013; 46(3):90-96.)

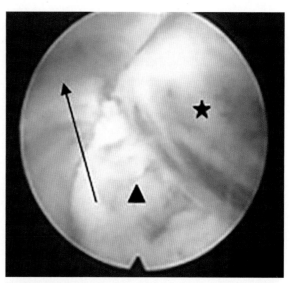

Fig. 4.26 Endoscopic view in the interlaminar approach demonstrating the herniated disc *(triangle)* when the nerve root *(star)* is pushed away by the working sheath *(long arrow)*. (From Hsu HT, Yang SS. Full-endoscopic interlaminar discectomy for herniation at L3–4 and L4–5: technical note. *Formosan J of Surg.* 2013;46(3):90-96.)

the endoscope is inserted, and the lateral aspect of the ligamentum flavum is removed with grasping forceps and Ellman electrodes. A puncture is then made on the lateral ligamentum flavum, and pressurized water is used to separate the dural sac from the ligamentum flavum. Under direct endoscopic view, the cannula is advanced through the puncture hole. The nerve root is then explored and identified via the cannula (Fig. 4.25). Once the shoulder portion of the nerve root is exposed, the nerve root is pushed internally with the nerve stripper. The external working sheath is then rotated to expose the herniated disc (Fig. 4.26). Grasping forceps are used to remove the damaged disc and degenerative tissues. The endoscope is angled to confirm removal and Ellman electrodes are used to finish the foraminaplasty. Decompression has been achieved once the nerve root is seen floating in the irrigation fluid (Fig. 4.27). Topical glucocorticoids are applied to reduce any nerve root inflammation. The L5–S1 level is ideal for this approach due to the wider interlaminar space. As a result, the interlaminar approach may have a faster

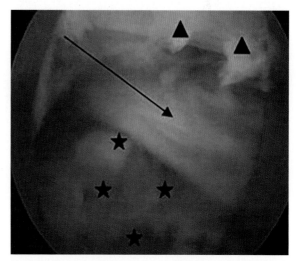

Fig. 4.27 Direct visualization of the complete resection of the herniated disc. The nerve root can be seen floating in the irrigation fluid. Ligamentum flavum *(triangles)*, nerve root *(long arrow)*, and margin of disc space *(stars)*. (From Hsu HT, Yang SS. Full-endoscopic interlaminar discectomy for herniation at L3–4 and L4–5: technical note. *Formosan J of Surg.* 2013;46(3):90-96.)

puncture orientation, shorter operation time, less radiation, and avoids the blockade by the crista iliaca.

ASSOCIATED COMPLICATIONS

The complications are similar to those for the other procedures. When comparing the transforaminal to the interlaminar approach, the transforaminal approach has a higher intraoperative radiation exposure, which can negatively affect the surgeon in the long term.

Conclusions

Minimally invasive discectomy techniques for the treatment of acute back pain caused by disc herniations offers the advantage over open discectomy of having fewer complications, less postoperative pain, less blood loss, fewer infections, and lower rates of reoperation.[56] Additionally, discectomy offers the advantage of resolving symptoms more quickly than conservative management and physical therapy, yet long term, one is not superior to the other.[3,5] Furthermore, minimally invasive techniques result in decreased hospital lengths of stay, less injury to surrounding structures, and lower acute care charges.[57] These minimally invasive techniques do have a much steeper learning curve that affect their outcomes; however, as the number of procedures performed continues to increase, physicians should become more familiar with the various approaches. Ultimately, such minimally invasive techniques offer an attractive treatment option for patients with acute herniated discs.

REFERENCES

1 Pengel LHM, Herbert RD, Maher CG, Refshauge KM. Acute low back pain: systematic review of its prognosis. *BMJ.* 2003; 327(7410):323.

2 Martin BI, Deyo RA, Mirza SK, et al. Expenditures and health status among adults with back and neck problems. *JAMA.* 2008;299(6):656-664.

3 Arts MP, Kuršumović A, Miller LE, et al. Comparison of treatments for lumbar disc herniation: systematic review with network meta-analysis. *Medicine (Baltimore).* 2019;98(7):e14410.

4 Ramaswami R, Ghogawala Z, Weinstein JN. Management of sciatica. *N Engl J Med.* 2017;376:1175-1177.

5 Peul WC, van Houwelingen HC, van den Hout WB, et al. Surgery versus prolonged conservative treatment for sciatica. *N Engl J Med.* 2007;356:2245-2256.

6 Peul WC, van den Hout WB, Brand R, Thomeer RTWM, Koes BW. Prolonged conservative care versus early surgery in patients with sciatica caused by lumbar disc herniation: two year results of a randomised controlled trial. *BMJ.* 2008;336:1355-1358.

7 Weinstein JN, Tosteson TD, Lurie JD, et al. Surgical vs nonoperative treatment for lumbar disk herniation: the Spine Patient Outcomes Research Trial (SPORT): a randomized trial. *JAMA.* 2006;296:2441-2450.

8 Carragee EJ, Spinnickie AO, Alamin TF, Paragioudakis SA. Prospective controlled study of limited versus subtotal posterior discectomy: short-term outcomes in patients with herniated lumbar intervertebral discs and large posterior anular defect. *Spine (Phila Pa 1976).* 2006;31:653-657.

9 Ambrossi GL, McGirt MJ, Sciubba DM, et al. Recurrent lumbar disc herniation after single-level lumbar discectomy: incidence and health care cost analysis. *Neurosurgery.* 2009;65:574-578; discussion 578.

10 McGirt MJ, Eustacchio S, Varga P, et al. A prospective cohort study of close interval computed tomography and magnetic resonance imaging after primary lumbar discectomy: factors associated with recurrent disc herniation and disc height loss. *Spine (Phila Pa 1976).* 2009;34:2044-2051.

11 Arts MP, Brand R, van den Akker ME, et al. Tubular diskectomy vs conventional microdiskectomy for the treatment of lumbar disk herniation: 2-year results of a double-blind randomized controlled trial. *Neurosurgery.* 2011;69:135-144; discussion 144.

12 Ran J, Hu Y, Zheng Z, et al. Comparison of discectomy versus sequestrectomy in lumbar disc herniation: a meta-analysis of comparative studies. *PLoS One.* 2015;10:e0121816.

13 Drazin D, Ugiliweneza B, Al-Khouja L, et al. Treatment of recurrent disc herniation: a systematic review. *Cureus.* 2016;8:e622.

14 Amin RM, Andrade NS, Neuman BJ. Lumbar disc herniation. *Curr Rev Musculoskelet Med.* 2017;10:507-516.

15 Kadow T, Sowa G, Vo N, Kang JD. Molecular basis of intervertebral disc degeneration and herniations: what are the important translational questions? *Clin Orthop Relat Res.* 2015;473: 1903-1912.

16 Kepler CK, Ponnappan RK, Tannoury CA, Risbud MV, Anderson DG. The molecular basis of intervertebral disc degeneration. *Spine J.* 2013;13:318-330.

17 Kalb S, Martirosyan NL, Kalani MY, Broc GG, Theodore N. Genetics of the degenerated intervertebral disc. *World Neurosurg.* 2012;77:491-501.

18 Urban JP, Roberts S. Degeneration of the intervertebral disc. *Arthritis Res Ther.* 2003;5:120-130.

19 Brayda-Bruno M, Tibiletti M, Ito K, et al. Advances in the diagnosis of degenerated lumbar discs and their possible clinical application. *Eur Spine J.* 2014;23(suppl 3):S315-S323.

20 Colombier P, Clouet J, Hamel O, Lescaudron L, Guicheux J. The lumbar intervertebral disc: from embryonic development to degeneration. *Joint Bone Spine.* 2014;81:125-129.

21 Mayer JE, Iatridis JC, Chan D, Qureshi SA, Gottesman O, Hecht AC. Genetic polymorphisms associated with intervertebral disc degeneration. *Spine J.* 2013;13:299-317.

22 Martirosyan NL, Patel AA, Carotenuto A, et al. Genetic alterations in intervertebral disc disease. *Front Surg.* 2016;3:59.

23 Janeczko L, Janeczko M, Chrzanowski R, Zielinski G. The role of polymorphisms of genes encoding collagen IX and XI in lumbar disc disease. *Neurol Neurochir Pol.* 2014;48:60-62.

24 Lama P, Le Maitre CL, Dolan P, Tarlton JF, Harding IJ, Adams MA. Do intervertebral discs degenerate before they herniate, or after? *Bone Joint J.* 2013;95-B:1127-1133.

25 Lotz JC, Chin JR. Intervertebral disc cell death is dependent on the magnitude and duration of spinal loading. *Spine (Phila Pa 1976)*. 2000;25:1477-1483.

26 Paul CPL, de Graaf M, Bisschop A, et al. Static axial overloading primes lumbar caprine intervertebral discs for posterior herniation. *PLoS One*. 2017;12:e0174278.

27 Lotz JC, Colliou OK, Chin JR, Duncan NA, Liebenberg E. Compression-induced degeneration of the intervertebral disc: an in vivo mouse model and finite-element study. *Spine (Phila Pa 1976)*. 1998;23:2493-2506.

28 Dydyk AM, Ngnitewe Massa R, Mesfin FB. Disc herination. In: *StatPearls*. 2022. Available at: https://www.ncbi.nlm.nih.gov/books/NBK441822/.

29 Park CH, Park ES, Lee SH, et al. Risk factors for early recurrence after transforaminal endoscopic lumbar disc decompression. *Pain Physician*. 2019;22:E133-E138.

30 Huang JS, Fan BK, Liu JM. Overview of risk factors for failed percutaneous transforaminal endoscopic discectomy in lumbar disc herniation. *Zhongguo Gu Shang*. 2019;32:186-189.

31 Waldman SD. Percutaneous Discectomy: Laser-Assisted Technique. In: Waldman SD, ed. *Atlas of Interventional Pain Management*. Philadelphia, PA: Elsevier; 2020:1038-1043.

32 Vucetic N, Svensson O. Physical signs in lumbar disc hernia. *Clin Orthop Relat Res*. 1996;(333):192-201.

33 Vroomen PC, de Krom MC, Wilmink JT, Kester AD, Knottnerus JA. Diagnostic value of history and physical examination in patients suspected of lumbosacral nerve root compression. *J Neurol Neurosurg Psychiatry*. 2002;72:630-634.

34 Kreiner DS, Hwang SW, Easa JE, et al. An evidence-based clinical guideline for the diagnosis and treatment of lumbar disc herniation with radiculopathy. *Spine J*. 2014;14:180-191.

35 Petersen T, Laslett M, Juhl C. Clinical classification in low back pain: best-evidence diagnostic rules based on systematic reviews. *BMC Musculoskelet Disord*. 2017;18:188.

36 Kim KY, Kim YT, Lee CS, Kang JS, Kim YJ. Magnetic resonance imaging in the evaluation of the lumbar herniated intervertebral disc. *Int Orthop*. 1993;17:241-244.

37 Messner A, Stelzeneder D, Trattnig S, et al. Does T2 mapping of the posterior annulus fibrosus indicate the presence of lumbar intervertebral disc herniation? A 3.0 Tesla magnetic resonance study. *Eur Spine J*. 2017;26:877-883.

38 Wong JJ, Côté P, Sutton DA, et al. Clinical practice guidelines for the noninvasive management of low back pain: a systematic review by the Ontario Protocol for Traffic Injury Management (OPTIMa) Collaboration. *Eur J Pain*. 2017;21:201-216.

39 Qaseem A, Wilt TJ, McLean RM, et al. Noninvasive treatments for acute, subacute, and chronic low back pain: a clinical practice guideline from the American College of Physicians. *Ann Intern Med*. 2017;166:514-530.

40 Chou R, Hashimoto R, Friedly J, et al. Epidural corticosteroid injections for radiculopathy and spinal stenosis: a systematic review and meta-analysis. *Ann Intern Med*. 2015;163:373-381.

41 Carette S, Leclaire R, Marcoux S, et al. Epidural corticosteroid injections for sciatica due to herniated nucleus pulposus. *N Engl J Med*. 1997;336:1634-1640.

42 Ackerman WE III, Ahmad M. The efficacy of lumbar epidural steroid injections in patients with lumbar disc herniations. *Anesth Analg*. 2007;104:1217-1222.

43 Wilson CA, Roffey DM, Chow D, Alkherayf F, Wai EK. A systematic review of preoperative predictors for postoperative clinical outcomes following lumbar discectomy. *Spine J*. 2016;16:1413-1422.

44 Shin BJ. Risk factors for recurrent lumbar disc herniations. *Asian Spine J*. 2014;8:211-215.

45 Huang W, Han Z, Liu J, Yu L, Yu X. Risk factors for recurrent lumbar disc herniation: a systematic review and meta-analysis. *Medicine (Baltimore)*. 2016;95:e2378.

46 Cinotti G, Roysam GS, Eisenstein SM, Postacchini F. Ipsilateral recurrent lumbar disc herniation. A prospective, controlled study. *J Bone Joint Surg Br*. 1998;80:825-832.

47 Kim KT, Park SW, Kim YB. Disc height and segmental motion as risk factors for recurrent lumbar disc herniation. *Spine (Phila Pa 1976)*. 2009;34:2674-2678.

48 Belykh E, Krutko AV, Baykov ES, Giers MB, Preul MC, Byvaltsev VA. Preoperative estimation of disc herniation recurrence after microdiscectomy: predictive value of a multivariate model based on radiographic parameters. *Spine J*. 2017;17:390-400.

49 Hegarty D, Shorten G. Multivariate prognostic modeling of persistent pain following lumbar discectomy. *Pain Physician*. 2012;15:421-434.

50 Atlas SJ, Deyo RA, Keller RB, et al. The Maine Lumbar Spine Study, Part II. 1-year outcomes of surgical and nonsurgical management of sciatica. *Spine (Phila Pa 1976)*. 1996;21:1777-1786.

51 Osterman H, Seitsalo S, Karppinen J, Malmivaara A. Effectiveness of microdiscectomy for lumbar disc herniation: a randomized controlled trial with 2 years of follow-up. *Spine (Phila Pa 1976)*. 2006;31:2409-2414.

52 Oba H, Takahashi J, Tsutsumimoto T, et al. Predictors of improvement in low back pain after lumbar decompression surgery: prospective study of 140 patients. *J Orthop Sci*. 2017;22:641-646.

53 Tschugg A, Lener S, Hartmann S, et al. Preoperative sport improves the outcome of lumbar disc surgery: a prospective monocentric cohort study. *Neurosurg Rev*. 2017;40:597-604.

54 Choi KC, Kim JS, Lee DC, Park CK. Outcome of decompression alone for foraminal/extraforaminal entrapment of L5 nerve root through Wiltse paraspinal approach. *Clin Spine Surg*. 2017;30:E1220-E1226.

55 Wiltse LL, Spencer CW. New uses and refinements of the paraspinal approach to the lumbar spine. *Spine (Phila Pa 1976)*. 1988;13:696-770.

56 Cahill KS, Levi AD, Cummock MD, Liao W, Wang MY. A comparison of acute hospital charges after tubular versus open microdiskectomy. *World Neurosurg*. 2013;80:208-212.

57 Phan K, Xu J, Schultz K, et al. Full-endoscopic versus microendoscopic and open discectomy: a systematic review and meta-analysis of outcomes and complications. *Clin Neurol Neurosurg*. 2017;154:1-12.

58 Waldman SD. In: *Atlas of Interventional Pain Management*. Philadelphia, PA: Elsevier; 2010:1031-1037.

59 Manchikanti L, Singh V, Falco FJE, et al. An updated review of automated percutaneous mechanical lumbar discectomy for the contained herniated lumbar disc. *Pain Physician*. 2013;16:SE151-SE184.

60 Waldman SD. In: *Atlas of Interventional Pain Management*. 5th ed. Philadelphia, PA: Elsevier; 2020:1044-1048.

61 Waldman SD. In: *Atlas of Interventional Pain*. 5th ed. Philadelphia, PA: Elsevier; 2020:1015-1024.

62 Nie H, Zeng J, Song Y, et al. Percutaneous endoscopic lumbar discectomy for L5-S1 disc herniation via an interlaminar approach versus a transforaminal approach: a prospective randomized controlled study with 2-year follow up. *Spine (Phila Pa 1976)*. 2016;41(suppl 19):B30-B37.

63 Choi KC, Kim JS, Ryu KS, Kang BU, Ahn Y, Lee SH. Percutaneous endoscopic lumbar discectomy for L5–S1 disc herniation: transforaminal versus interlaminar approach. *Pain Physician.* 2013;16:547-556.

64 Hoogland T, Schubert M, Miklitz B, Ramirez A. Transforaminal posterolateral endoscopic discectomy with or without the combination of a low-dose chymopapain: a prospective randomized study in 280 consecutive cases. *Spine (Phila Pa 1976).* 2006;31:E890-E897.

65 Mariscalco MW, Yamashita T, Steinmetz MP, Krishnaney AA, Lieberman IH, Mroz TE. Radiation exposure to the surgeon during open lumbar microdiscectomy and minimally invasive microdiscectomy: a prospective, controlled trial. *Spine (Phila Pa 1976).* 2011;36:255-260.

66 Ahn Y, Lee SH, Park WM, Lee HY, Shin SW, Kan HY. Percutaneous endoscopic lumbar discectomy for recurrent disc herniation: surgical technique, outcome, and prognostic factors of 43 consecutive cases. *Spine (Phila Pa 1976).* 2004;29:E326-E332.

Chapter 5

Interspinous Spacer

Ryan Budwany and Yeshvant Navalgund

Introduction

The interspinous spacer procedure provides patients with a minimally invasive solution that is designed to deliver long-term relief from the leg and back pain associated with lumbar spinal stenosis (LSS). The procedure uses a small, titanium alloy spacer that serves as an extension blocker designed to relieve pressure on the affected nerves. This helps minimize the effects of spinal degeneration while fully preserving the patient's anatomy.[1]

Indications

The interspinous spacer indirect decompression is indicated for treatment of patients with neurogenic claudication from moderate degenerative LSS, in a stable spine, with no greater than grade 1 spondylolisthesis. The ideal candidates are patients who can relieve their symptoms with flexion or sitting. The indications for the interspinous spacer procedure are very specific: mild to moderate central, lateral, and/or foraminal spinal stenosis with neurogenic claudication.

Contraindications

1. Cauda equina syndrome
2. Severe weakness
3. Significant scoliosis
4. Acute fractures of the spinous process or vertebral body
5. Greater than grade 1 spondylolisthesis
6. Prior fusion or decompression at the indicated level
7. Severe osteoporosis (DEXA scan equivalent greater than 2.5 standard deviation)
8. Active local or systemic infection
9. Allergy to titanium

In addition to the contraindications listed here, there are anatomical considerations to be aware of.[2]

"KISSING SPINE"

Where spinous processes are in very close approximation (Fig. 5.1), or in contact (i.e., "kissing"), this anatomy may result in increased difficulty in placement of the cannula.

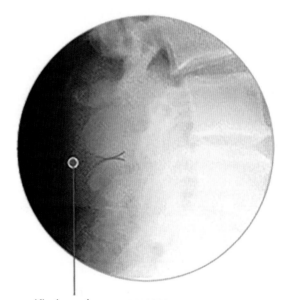

Kissing spinous processes

Fig. 5.1 Kissing spinous processes. (Courtesy of Boston Scientific Corporation.)

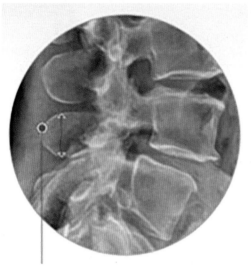

Thin spinous process

Fig. 5.2 Thin spinous processes. (Courtesy of Boston Scientific Corporation.)

THIN, OR "GRACILE" SPINOUS PROCESSES

When a spinous process is unusually thin (Fig. 5.2), or measures less than 20 mm in superior-inferior dimension, the likelihood of a postoperative spinous process fracture may be increased.

Perioperative Considerations

PATIENT SELECTION

The ideal candidates for the interspinous spacer procedure are patients who can relieve their symptoms with flexion or sitting. The procedure is appropriate for treating various types of spinal stenosis, including central, lateral, and foraminal (or combinations thereof) with neurogenic claudication.

Preoperative Considerations

Table 5.1 describes some important aspects of the procedure setup.

PROCEDURE

The device is implanted utilizing the tools provided in a sterile tool kit (Fig. 5.3).

1. Patient position should be in the prone position with optimally flexed lumbar spine (Fig. 5.4).
2. Identify level to be treated.
   Use dilator assembly, hemostat, spinal needle, or K-wire to confirm midline and axial position (Fig. 5.5). Single or biplane fluoroscopy may be used.
3. Identify the appropriate surgical level and accurate midline position using a spinal needle, dilator assembly, or scalpel with anterioposterior (AP) and lateral fluoroscopy.
   After confirmation of the surgical level, create a 12–15 mm midline incision at the operable level with a scalpel (Fig. 5.6). Dissect to the depth of the supraspinous ligament (SSL). Advance the blade with AP and lateral fluoroscopy to produce a longitudinal split of the SSL at midline (Fig. 5.7).
4. Advance the guide dilator manually and if necessary, with a mallet, until the distal tip approaches

TABLE 5.1	Procedure Setup
Anesthesia	Mild to moderate sedation Deep sedation or general anesthesia should be avoided unless performed with nerve monitoring
Positioning	Prone position with flattened or minimized lumbar lordosis No pressure on the belly or chest for ease of breathing for the patient
Antimicrobial actions	Appropriate antibiotic is given before the start of the procedure The target area is scrubbed with 2%–3% chlorhexidine/70% isopropyl alcohol solution and allowed to dry for 3 min Full surgical drapes are used, and the target skin area is covered with an antimicrobial incise drape (e.g., Ioban)

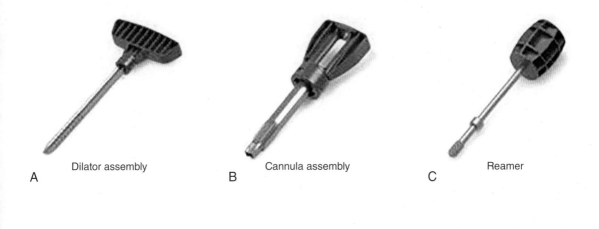

A Dilator assembly B Cannula assembly C Reamer

D Interspinous gauge E Inserter F Driver

Fig. 5.3 Sterile tool kit. (Courtesy of Boston Scientific Corporation.)

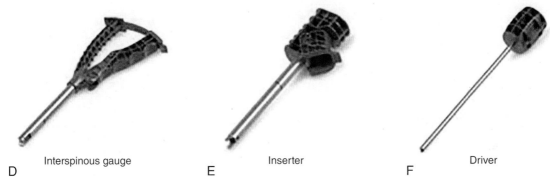

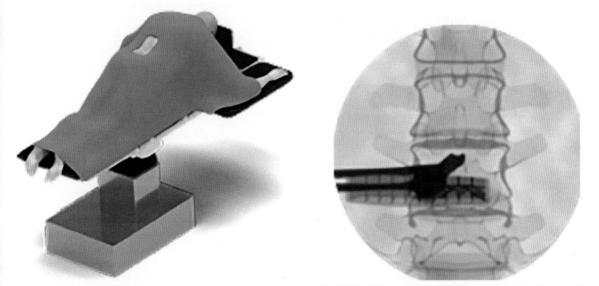

Fig. 5.4 Patient positioning: flexed. (Courtesy of Boston Scientific Corporation.)

Fig. 5.5 Identify treatment level. (Courtesy of Boston Scientific Corporation.)

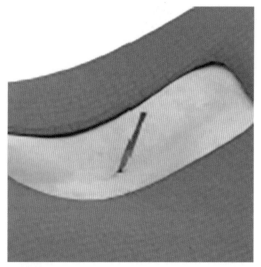

Fig. 5.6 Skin incision. (Courtesy of Boston Scientific Corporation.)

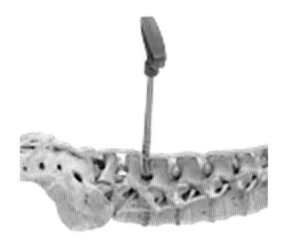

Fig. 5.8 Dilator assembly placement. (Courtesy of Boston Scientific Corporation.)

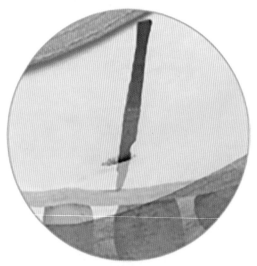

Fig. 5.7 Longitudinal split of supraspinous ligament. (Courtesy of Boston Scientific Corporation.)

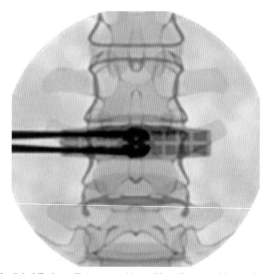

Fig. 5.9 A/P view: dilator assembly position. (Courtesy of Boston Scientific Corporation.)

the dorsal facet shadow (spinal laminar junction). This should be performed in the lateral fluoroscopic view to avoid dural injury.

Place the dilator assembly into the treatment site at midline and confirm position with AP fluoroscopy. Advance the dilator assembly manually and with the assistance of a mallet, until the distal tip approaches the dorsal aspect of the facet shadow (Fig. 5.8). Use AP

fluoroscopy to confirm midline placement (Fig. 5.9). Utilize instrument depth markers and lateral fluoroscopy to verify depth (Fig. 5.10). Once midline position and depth are confirmed, unlock and remove the dilator assembly handle, leaving only the dilator.

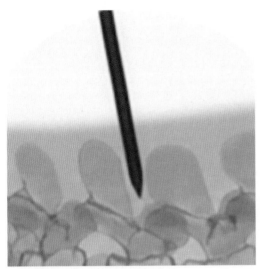

Fig. 5.10 Lateral view: dilator assembly position. (Courtesy of Boston Scientific Corporation.)

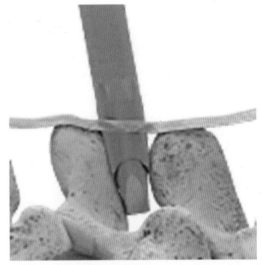

Fig. 5.12 Cannula position detail. (Courtesy of Boston Scientific Corporation.)

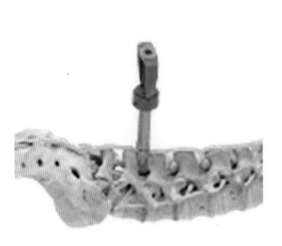

Fig. 5.11 Cannula assembly placement. (Courtesy of Boston Scientific Corporation.)

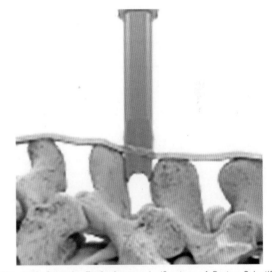

Fig. 5.13 Cannula final placement. (Courtesy of Boston Scientific Corporation.)

5. Advance the cannula assembly manually, or using a mallet, taking care to ensure the dilator does not advance further. Advance the cannula assembly until the distal tip reaches the dorsal aspect of the facet shadow and is firmly seated between the adjacent spinous processes (Fig. 5.11).

Use lateral fluoroscopy to monitor depth of insertion. When position is confirmed, remove dilator. Unlock and remove the cannula assembly handle, ultimately leaving only the outer cannula (hereinafter referred to as cannula). Confirm the position of the cannula to flank the spinous process above and below (Fig. 5.12).

6. Use the interspinous reamer to create space between the spinous processes to allow room for the implanted spacer (Figs. 5.13–5.15).

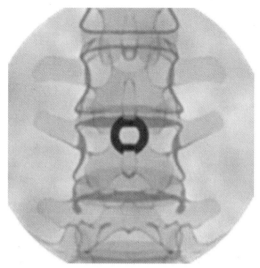

Fig. 5.14 A/P confirmation of cannula placement and midline trajectory. (Courtesy of Boston Scientific Corporation.)

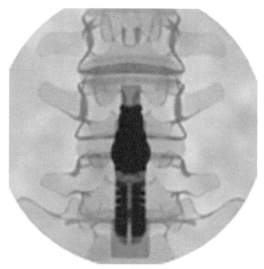

Fig. 5.16 Interspinous gauge: anterioposterior Ferguson superior aspect. (Courtesy of Boston Scientific Corporation.)

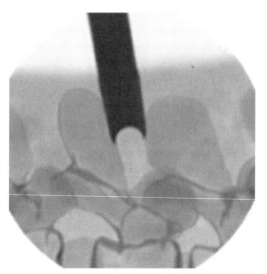

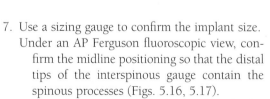

Fig. 5.15 Lateral confirmation of cannula depth. (Courtesy of Boston Scientific Corporation.)

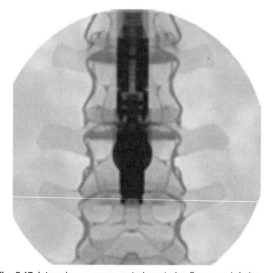

Fig. 5.17 Interspinous gauge: anterioposterior Ferguson inferior aspect. (Courtesy of Boston Scientific Corporation.)

7. Use a sizing gauge to confirm the implant size. Under an AP Ferguson fluoroscopic view, confirm the midline positioning so that the distal tips of the interspinous gauge contain the spinous processes (Figs. 5.16, 5.17).
8. Insert the implant with the implant loader (Fig. 5.18)
9. Deploy the implant.

10. Use AP and lateral fluoroscopy to confirm deployment of the implant to flank the superior and inferior spinous processes (Figs. 5.19, 5.20).
11. Advance deployed implant to at least the anterior half of the spinous processes.
12. Release the implant. Confirm with imaging (Figs. 5.21, 5.22)

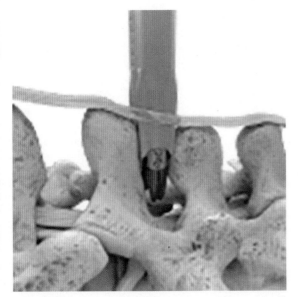

Fig. 5.18 Minimum insertion depth. (Courtesy of Boston Scientific Corporation.)

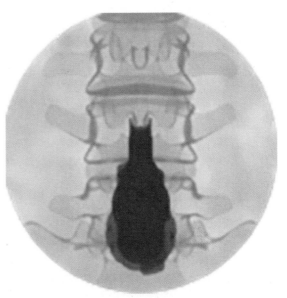

Fig. 5.20 Verify containment of spinous processes. (Courtesy of Boston Scientific Corporation.)

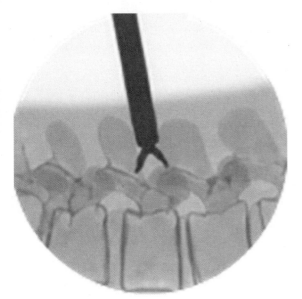

Fig. 5.19 Verify depth under lateral fluoroscopy. (Courtesy of Boston Scientific Corporation.)

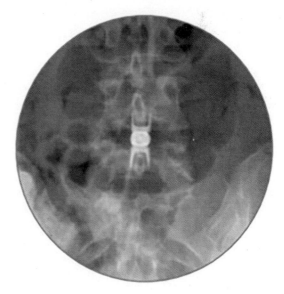

Fig. 5.21 Anterioposterior verification of implant position. (Courtesy of Boston Scientific Corporation.)

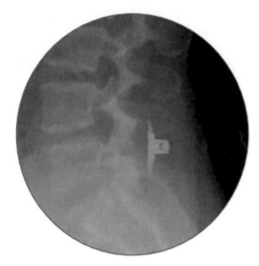

Fig. 5.22 Lateral verification of implant position. (Courtesy of Boston Scientific Corporation.)

Postoperative Considerations

Table 5.2 describes some important aspects of the post procedure care.

Management, If Failed

Complications associated with the interspinous spacer procedure can include displacement of the device with worsening spondylolisthesis.

Therapeutic failures should prompt the clinician to investigate other causes of the patient's symptoms, including other potentially affected adjacent spinal segments. In rare circumstances, the device will require removal and the patient should be referred for surgical intervention.

Postoperative infections can occur. Treatment necessitates removal of the device and appropriate antibiotic treatment. In most instances, a new device can be placed once the infection is cleared. Vigilance should be exercised to monitor patients closely postoperatively to ensure early detection of infection.

Removal of the device can be done either by an open procedure or under fluoroscopic guidance using the aforementioned dilation techniques. Once the inserter is locked in place, the driver is placed and gently rotated until it engages the implant. Continue to rotate counterclockwise until the implant is completely disengaged from the spinal processes and can be withdrawn.

Clinical Pearls

- Two contiguous levels can be performed, but the most symptomatic level should be treated first to ensure adequate decompression.
- Do not deploy the dilator too deep. If it is too deep, you will have difficulty deploying the implant. Additionally, be precise and meticulous about your alignment.
- Ensure throughout the procedure that your placement is optimal. This is going to allow for ease of deployment of the implant.

TABLE 5.2	Postprocedural Care
Acute recovery	Observation in recovery area until sedation wears off Brief neurological examination is performed before discharge
Discharge instructions	No need for postprocedure antibiotic coverage Patient can ambulate freely once at home Postprocedure pain should ease up in a few days
Follow-up care	Patient should return in 2 weeks to evaluate the extent of symptom relief At times, optimal functional improvement requires a course of physical therapy for muscle strengthening and conditioning Physical therapy should not be considered until at least 8 weeks postprocedure in order to allow the device to scar into place, thus minimizing the chance for dislodgement A final assessment of patient improvement may not be feasible until a few months postprocedure

- Patients with scoliosis can be treated, but it is imperative that the Cobb angle at the level to be treated is no greater than 10 degrees.
- The interspinous gauge should not be over- or under-deployed, as oversizing can cause increased pain or fracture at the site and undersizing can inhibit adequate decompression of the targeted treatment level.
- Perioperative antibiotics should be administered similar to the case of other implantable devices.
- Patients who have undergone a fusion where adjacent levels above or below the fusion have developed symptomatic stenosis may still be candidates for this procedure. Additionally, patients with previously placed implantable devices like intrathecal pumps or spinal cord stimulators that have developed symptomatic lumbar stenosis also may be candidates. Avoid patients who have undergone a hemilaminectomy, as the integrity of the spinous process is less and may predispose to fracture.

REFERENCES

1. Boston Scientific. *The Vertiflex Procedure*. Available at: https://www.bostonscientific.com/en-US/medical-specialties/pain-management/the-vertiflex-procedure.html.
2. Boston Scientific. Vertiflex Superion Indirect Decompression System: Instructions for Use. Valenica, CA; 2020.

Chapter 6

Minimally Invasive Lumbar Decompression

Ryan Budwany and Yeshvant Navalgund

Introduction

Minimally invasive lumbar decompression (MILD) is an image-guided approach used in the treatment of symptomatic lumbar central spinal stenosis. This procedure is a good option for patients who are not responsive to conservative or injection therapy and either do not want an open surgical decompression or are not good surgical candidates. Lumbar spinal stenosis (LSS) is a degenerative disease of the aging spine. LSS is the most common indication for spinal surgery in patients above the age of 65.[1]

Indication

The MILD procedure is indicated for patients with symptomatic central LSS due to ligamentum flavum hypertrophy. It is not meant for patients with symptoms due to lateral recess spinal stenosis. It is also not indicated if stenosis is due to any cause other than ligamentum flavum hypertrophy (e.g., anterolisthesis or disc protrusion). Indications and contraindications are summarized in Table 6.1.

TABLE 6.1 Indications and Contraindications for MILD Procedure	
Indications	**Contraindications**
• Ligamentum hypertrophy preferably >4 mm² • Central spinal stenosis • Symptoms of neurogenic claudication • No sensory or motor defect	• Coagulopathy • Surgery at that level • Severe scoliosis • True allergy to dye • Only back pain

MILD, Minimally invasive lumbar decompression

Patient Selection

Patient selection is the most important part of the MILD procedure (Table 6.2). The patient should have symptomatic central LSS from ligamentum flavum hypertrophy (Fig. 6.1).

Setup

Table 6.3 describes some important aspects of the procedure setup.

Procedure

1. Obtain an anterioposterior fluoroscopic view of the lumbar spine with the spinous process midway between the pedicles.
2. Three straight lines are drawn:
   - One in the middle (over the spinous processes)
   - Two connecting the medial side of the pedicles on each side (Fig. 6.2)
3. Ideally, the insertion point is usually one and one-half to two vertebral levels below the target space, in the paramedian plane between the two lines initially drawn on the patient in the previous step.
4. Provide cutaneous analgesia with a 25-gauge needle, then further anesthetize the cannula tract with a 22-gauge 3.5 inch spinal needle to the lower lamina, including the laminar periosteum.
5. Obtain epidural space access. The epidural needle should be placed in the most cephalad part of the interlaminar space with the intent to obtain ipsilateral dye spread.

TABLE 6.2	Patient Selection Factors
Primary indication	Neurogenic claudication in the presence of radiologically proven ligamentum flavum hypertrophy
Neurogenic claudication symptoms	• Pain • Numbness • Weakness • Tingling in low back, buttocks, and legs initiated by standing, walking, or lumbar extension that is relieved by sitting or forward flexion.
Symptom characteristics	Symptoms do not follow a dermatomal pattern (a hallmark of foraminal or lateral recess stenosis), but the two distinct etiologies can coexist The symptoms tend to be symmetrical, usually above the knee; this proximal distribution helps to symptomatically differentiate lumbar stenosis from vascular claudication[3]
Physical examination	Unremarkable; the presence of sensory or motor deficits should prompt surgical evaluation
Imaging	Imaging is required for the definite diagnosis of LSS[4] A systemic review found CT or MRI equally accurate in the diagnosis of LSS[5] MRI is preferred as ligament hypertrophy can be easily measured
Radiological criteria for spinal stenosis	There are several criteria used, but anterioposterior spinal canal diameter of <10 mm or an area of <70 mm^2 is generally considered diagnostic[6]
Diagnostic criteria used in various MILD trials	• Neurogenic claudication for at least 3 months • Ligamentum flavum thickness of >2.5 mm • Anterolisthesis of 5 mm or less • Absence of spinal instability

LSS, Lumbar spinal stenosis

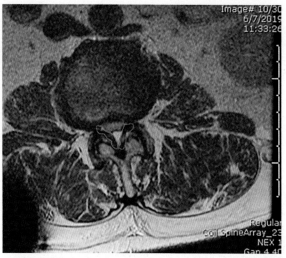

Fig. 6.1 Thickened ligamentum flavum outlined in *red* on axial view MRI lumbar spine.

TABLE 6.3	Procedure Setup
Anesthesia	Mild to moderate sedation Deep sedation or general anesthesia should be avoided unless performed with nerve monitoring
Positioning	Prone position with flattened or minimized lumbar lordosis No pressure on the belly or chest for ease of breathing for the patient
Antimicrobial actions	Appropriate antibiotic is given before the start of the procedure The target area is scrubbed with 2%–3% chlorhexidine/70% isopropyl alcohol solution, which is allowed to dry for 3 minutes Full surgical drapes are used, and the target skin area is covered with an antimicrobial incise drape (e.g., Ioban)

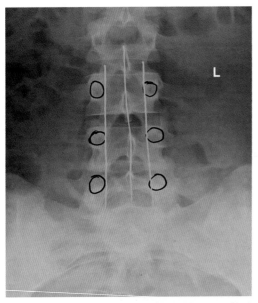

Fig. 6.2 Three *green lines* drawn define the working area. *Black circles* outline the pedicles.

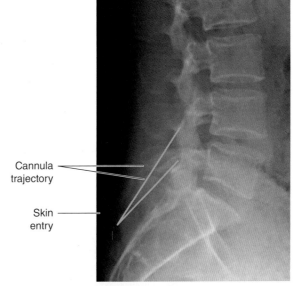

Fig. 6.3 Planning trajectory using lateral view. *Green lines* demonstrate working cannula trajectory *(double arrows point to cannula)*. Skin entry *(single black arrow)* is at the lower portion of the lamina.

6. After a skin stab, a 6-gauge working cannula via use of the trocar is inserted to the lower lamina.
7. Lateral fluoroscopic guidance is used to ensure that it is not placed too deep (which will result in a large dural tear) (Figs. 6.3, 6.4).
8. Obtain a contralateral oblique view (Fig. 6.5).
   • The optimal view is one that allows laminar outlines to appear the thickest and the crispest. This angle is usually around 40–45 degrees contralateral oblique.

• Cephalocaudal tilting may be required to obtain the optimal working view.
• The intention is to get the X-ray beam perfectly parallel to the ipsilateral lamina.
• The configuration of epidurogram seen in this view confirms the location of the stenosis and serves as a safety check and constant reminder of the plane that should not be violated. Therefore, it is important to maintain the epidurogram by frequently injecting dye throughout the procedure.

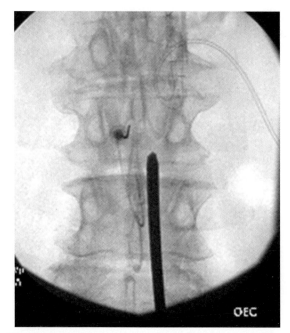

Fig. 6.4 Anterioposterior view of working cannula placed at the lower lamina.

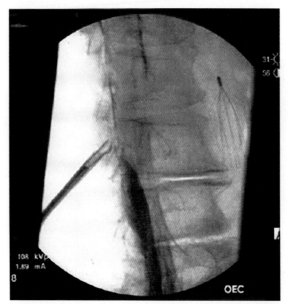

Fig. 6.5 Contralateral oblique photo shows posterior to anterior plane. Contrast media marks epidural space, and position of mild Tissue Sculptor tip (left side of photo) is shown relative to bony and soft tissue landmarks.

- The improvement in the contour of the epidurogram is one of the endpoints of this procedure.

Key Safety Note: The epidurogram represents the plane that should not be violated with any instrument during the procedure.

9. Using manual control and imaging guidance, advance the tissue access device cephalad at an acute angle to the spine with gentle but firm pressure. Direct toward the dorsal surface of the spinal lamina of the adjacent vertebral segment, inferior to the interlaminar space and lateral to the spinous process (Fig. 6.6).

10. After the working cannula is in place, a portal stabilizer device is used to stabilize the cannula (Fig. 6.7). The device grips the cannula, thus preventing it from inadvertently advancing during the procedure.

11. The trocar is removed and another piece from the kit, the depth guide device, is placed over

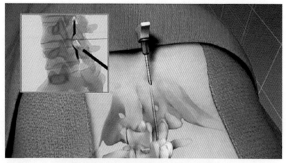

Fig. 6.6 Tissue access device placement.

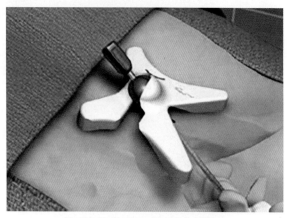

Fig. 6.7 Positioning with portal stabilizer.

it. The depth guide limits the risk of subsequent instruments unintentionally being pushed too far in through the cannula.

12. A bone rongeur is advanced through the portal under fluoroscopic guidance.

13. The space between the laminae is opened by snipping away bone, first from the lower edge of the upper lamina and then by flipping the rongeur and snipping from the upper edge of the lower lamina (Fig. 6.8).

14. This process also loosens the ligamentum flavum attachment from the lower lamina, making it easier to sculpt.

15. The interlaminar space is opened by repeating these steps more medially and laterally, thus creating a good opening. Fluoroscopic guidance should be used throughout.

16. The lines drawn at the start of the procedure (see Fig. 6.2) are helpful to avoid angling the rongeur too far medially or laterally. The trigger of the bone rongeur should be pulled slowly in case one needs to stop the bite at any time.

17. It is important to be patient and judiciously remove small amounts of bone with any bite. The depth guide device may need adjustments to gain access to the deeper part of the laminae.

18. Once enough space has been created, the tissue sculptor is inserted through the portal. The tissue sculptor end is shaped like an ice cream scoop and is specifically designed with the cutting edge on the inner lip. It only scrapes tissue when employing an upward scooping movement (Fig. 6.9).

19. The stroke starts from the lower lamina and ends at the upper lamina, at which point the trigger of the tissue sculptor is pulled, which resects the ligament flavum and collects the resected tissue.

20. All tissue bites should be performed with live fluoroscopy in the contralateral oblique view. The movement is repeated a few times, and then the sculptor is retracted and any resected tissue is removed by pushing it out of the sculptor with the thumb trigger. The procedure is repeated until enough tissue has been removed.

21. Adequate tissue removal is confirmed via visualization of straightening and thickening of the epidurogram outline as an indication that the spinal space has opened up (Figs. 6.10, 6.11).

22. Additional ligaments may need to be removed either medially and/or laterally and this procedure should be guided by MRI.

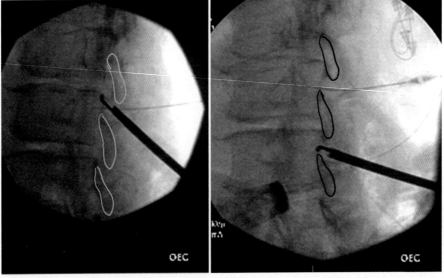

Fig. 6.8 Bone rongeur in *(left)* contralateral oblique view of laminar border in green in cephalad position and *(right)* contralateral oblique view of laminar border in black in caudad position.

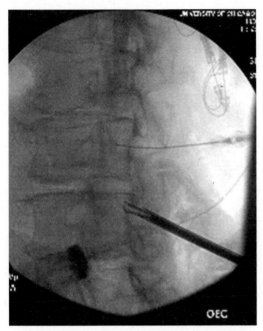

Fig. 6.9 Tissue sculptor in contralateral oblique view.

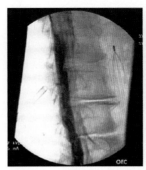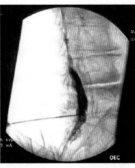

Fig. 6.10 Changes in epidurogram demonstrate post procedure free flowing contrast on the left and constricted flow of contrast pre procedure on the right.

23. This procedure removes only the dorsal part of the ligament flavum, leaving the ventral part intact. The amount of tissue removed is not related to the extent of pain relief obtained, and it is not necessary to measure the volume of tissue removed.

24. Once the epidural space has opened enough, as seen on the epidurogram, the working cannula is removed.

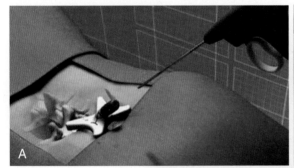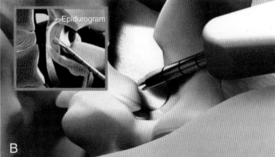

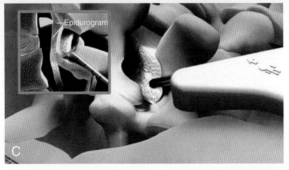

Fig. 6.11 MILD tissue sculpting. (A) insertion of tissue sculptor, (B) approach to tissue, (C) clearing of tissue.

25. The epidural needle is removed partially and redirected to obtain epidural space access in the contralateral side.
26. The working cannula is placed on the other side and the whole procedure is repeated.
27. Once the treatment of spinal stenosis at one level is complete, the procedure may be repeated at an additional interlaminar level.
28. The procedure may be performed at two adjacent spinal levels via use of a single skin puncture if the patient's physique is amenable.
29. This dual-level approach requires performing the procedure on the ipsilateral side at two interlaminar spaces and then removing the portal prior to insertion on the contralateral side.
30. Once the procedure endpoint has been achieved, the cannula is removed, and the skin is closed with skin glue and Steri-Strips. Suturing is not generally required.

Postprocedure Care

Table 6.4 describes some important aspects of postprocedure care.

Complications

There is always a risk of infection, bleeding, or nerve damage. No such complication has been reported in published studies. There is risk of a large dural tear, but this also has not been reported.

Procedure Effectiveness

Several observational and few randomized studies have shown that the procedure provides durable relief and meaningful improvements in functional status in properly selected patients. The 2-year follow-up of patients enrolled in the MiDAS ENCORE trial showed a mean improvement in visual analog scale score of 3.6 points and a mean improvement in Oswestry Disability Index of 22.7 points.[7] A systematic review found that although the procedure seems to be relatively safe, the current evidence on MILD for the treatment of symptomatic LSS is of low quality and suffers from a risk of bias.[8] In addition, no postprocedure imaging study has been completed that has demonstrably correlated symptomatic improvements with improvements in the extent of central spinal stenosis. Though MILD has demonstrated efficacy compared with lumbar epidural steroid injections, the procedure has not been compared head-to-head with surgery.[9,10]

Management, If Failed

If the MILD procedure fails to completely decompress central spinal stenosis, the patient should be referred for traditional spinal decompression surgery.

Clinical Pearls

- Ensure symptoms are related to central spinal stenosis.
- Insert the epidural needle high in the interlaminar space, out of way of other instruments.
- Ensure an ipsilateral epidurogram for each side.
- Ensure adequate opening of the interlaminar space using a bone rongeur.
- Remove enough tissue to improve the contour of the epidurogram.

TABLE 6.4	Postprocedure Care
Acute recovery	Observation in recovery area until sedation wears off Brief neurological examination is performed before discharge
Discharge instructions	No need for postprocedure antibiotic coverage Patient can ambulate freely once at home Postprocedure pain should ease up in a few days
Follow-up care	Patient should return in 2 weeks to evaluate the extent of symptom relief At times, optimal functional improvement requires a course of physical therapy for muscle strengthening and conditioning A final assessment of patient improvement may not be feasible until a few months postprocedure

REFERENCES

1. Jain S, Deer T, Sayed D, et al. Minimally invasive lumbar decompression: a review of indications, techniques, efficacy, and safety. *Pain Management.* 2020;10(5):331-348.
2. Kim YU, Park JY, Kim DH, et al. The role of the ligamentum flavum area as a morphological parameter of lumbar central spinal stenosis. *Pain Physician.* 2017;20(3):E419-E424.
3. Nadeau M, Rosas-Arellano M, Gurr K, et al. The reliability of differentiating neurogenic claudication from vascular claudication based on symptomatic presentation. *Can J Surg.* 2013;56:372-377.
4. de Schepper EIT, Overdevest GM, Suri P, et al. Diagnosis of lumbar spinal stenosis: an updated systematic review of the accuracy of diagnostic tests. *Spine (Phila Pa 1976).* 2013;38(8):E469-E481.
5. de Graaf I, Prak A, Bierma-Zeinstra S, Thomas S, Peul W, Koes B. Diagnosis of lumbar spinal stenosis: a systematic review of the accuracy of diagnostic tests. *Spine (Phila Pa 1976).* 2006;31(10):1168-1176.
6. Steurer J, Roner S, Gnannt R, Hodler J, LumbSten Research Collaboration. Quantitative radiologic criteria for the diagnosis of lumbar spinal stenosis: a systematic literature review. *BMC Musculoskelet Disord.* 2011;12:175.
7. Staats PS, Benyamin RM, MiDAS ENCORE Investigators. MiDAS ENCORE: randomized controlled clinical trial report of 6-month results. *Pain Physician.* 2016;19(2):25-38.
8. Kreiner DS, MacVicar J, Duszynski B, et al. The MILD procedure: a systematic review of the current literature. *Pain Med Malden Mass.* 2014;15:196-220.
9. Brown LL. A double-blind, randomized, prospective study of epidural steroid injection vs. the mild® procedure in patients with symptomatic lumbar spinal stenosis. *Pain Pract.* 2012;12(5):333-341.
10. Benyamin RM, Staats PS, MiDAS ENCORE I. Mild® is an effective treatment for lumbar spinal stenosis with neurogenic claudication: MiDAS ENCORE randomized controlled trial. *Pain Physician.* 2016;19(4):229-242.

Chapter 7

Cervical and Lumbar Foraminotomy for the Management of Chronic Radicular Back Pain

Jarod Speer, Marianne Tanios, Maher Kodsy, and Alaa Abd-Elsayed

Introduction

Foraminal stenosis and herniated discs are common pathologies seen in primary care and chronic pain clinics. The radicular pain caused by these anatomic abnormalities may be difficult to manage medically, and invasive surgical interventions can result in significant complications. Typically, discectomy and spinal fusion are considered gold standard techniques to treat radiculopathic pain. These operations require general anesthesia, postoperative recovery, and can result in limited postoperative spinal range of motion. By contrast, foraminotomy serves as a safe, minimally invasive alternative that is performed under local anesthesia and can preserve intervertebral range of motion.[1,2] Foraminotomy is a particularly appealing option for patients who fail conservative medical management and are poor surgical candidates. In appropriate patients, foraminotomy is an interventional option to decompress nerve roots and provide significant radiculopathic symptom relief and pain control.[3]

In cases of cervical radiculopathy, two approaches with comparable results are often employed; full-endoscopic posterior cervical foraminotomy (FE-PCF), and microscopic posterior cervical foraminotomy (MI-PCF).[4] The appropriately trained pain management specialist can utilize a minimally invasive keyhole transforaminal approach and facilitate nonfusion, nondiscectomy foraminotomy; minimizing blood loss, surgical trauma, and loss of intervertebral range of motion.[1,5,6]

Indications

INDICATIONS FOR CERVICAL FORAMINOTOMY

Unilateral cervical radiculopathy and resistant cervical neuropathic pain secondary to cervical foraminal stenosis are the primary indications for cervical foraminotomy; however, consideration for foraminotomy is generally reserved for patients who fail to respond to conservative management for a minimum of 6 weeks.[2] Conservative management generally includes immobilization, massage, physical therapy, cervical steroid injections, and oral medications.[6] In the event of conservative management failure, posterior cervical foraminotomy (PCF) may be considered if the patient has radicular symptoms in the absence of central spinal cord compression.[2,6] In addition, cervical radiculopathy should generally be secondary to lateral or foraminal disc herniation narrowing foraminal space, osteophytic nerve compression, or primary foraminal stenosis,[7-9] and compressive disease should be limited to two or less unilateral cervical levels.[9] Lateral disc herniation leading to narrowing cervical foramina is critical, as cervical myelin must not be mobilized toward the midline.[8,10] For consideration of foraminotomy for cervical radiculopathy, nerve pain symptoms should be consistent with anatomic pathology seen on imaging studies.[2,5] Patients may require repeat foraminotomy following previous endoscopic foraminotomy if symptoms recur; however, consideration for repeat foraminotomy requires evaluation of each patient's specific circumstances, and consideration of the factors that led to treatment failure.

INDICATIONS FOR LUMBAR FORAMINOTOMY

Like cervical foraminotomy, operative intervention for lumbar radiculopathy and neuropathic pain is typically reserved for patients who fail to respond to conservative management. In general, we consider indications for cervical and lumber foraminotomy to be similar; however, neurogenic claudication, leg pain, and symptoms of sciatica may be more common in lumbar foraminal stenosis and may serve as indications for lumber foraminotomy.

Contraindications

Contraindications to foraminotomy serve to protect patients from poor outcomes and assist the interventionalist in risk-mitigation strategies. As is the case with most operative interventions, active infection, previous spinal surgery with hardware, and operative field tumor serve as direct contraindications to foraminotomy.[11] Spinal segmental instability[11] and significant anatomic abnormalities including significant chronic kyphosis, severe degenerative changes, and evidence of spinal cord compression are all contraindications to foraminotomy.[2,12] Significant vertebral body pathology including fracture, and concomitant myelopathy are also contraindications to foraminotomy.[2]

Preoperative Considerations

An individualized approach to perioperative evaluation should be employed to optimize patient outcomes with careful individual considerations of operative indications and contraindications present in each case. Preoperative evaluation with radiologic studies, particularly MRI is essential. MRI evaluation serves to characterize foraminal size, degree of disease progression, and presence of concomitant contraindications to foraminotomy.

In general, a posterior approach is most often preferred over an anterior approach for cervical foraminotomy, as an anterior approach carries an increased risk of visceral injury and recurrent laryngeal nerve palsy as well as worse cosmetic outcomes.[13] PCF postoperative

outcomes can be further optimized by taking special care to characterize biomechanical measurements preoperatively to determine the intervertebral range of motion, facet joint space, and intervertebral disc pressure.[14]

For lumbar foraminotomy, a posterolateral approach may be used for foraminal and extra foraminal stenosis, a lateral approach is preferred for recess stenosis with or without herniation, and a transforaminal approach is used for central spinal stenosis.[15]

Irrespective of location however, the key to successful operative management of disc herniation and foraminal stenosis is exposure of the target nerve root. Therefore, careful analysis of MRI studies should be undertaken to identify the position of the working cannula by first identifying anatomic landmarks; caudal pedicle, disc space, and the posterior wall of the cranial and caudal vertebrae.[15] The procedural needle trajectory will be planned using preoperative image studies.[16] With appropriate preoperative planning and patient selection, the likelihood of positive foraminotomy outcomes can be optimized.

Physical Examination

Patients should be thoroughly evaluated prior to consideration for operative intervention. Typically, appropriate patients demonstrate unilateral radiculopathy, pain, and dermatomal paresthesias. In more severe cases patients may have depressed deep tendon reflexes (in cases of lumbar radiculopathy), and unilateral weakness.

Specific physical examination maneuvers may be utilized to differentiate the cause of pain in a patient experiencing radicular symptoms before imaging studies are obtained. The Spurling maneuver, a foraminal compression test, is particularly specific for a diagnosis of cervical radiculopathy.[17] Traction or neck distraction has been shown to be highly specific for radiculopathy as well if these maneuvers result in an improvement in symptoms.[17] The combination of suspicious patient history and symptomatology with positive provocative and relieving examination maneuvers should prompt imaging evaluation.

Radiologic Examination

MRI is the imaging study of choice, and it should be utilized preoperatively to confirm spinal stenosis, herniated disc, or foraminal narrowing or defect. Preoperative imaging will also guide procedural planning.[15,16]

Procedure

LUMBAR FORAMINOTOMY: TRANSFORAMINAL APPROACH[15]

To perform lumbar foraminotomy, the patient is placed in a comfortable prone position under C-arm fluoroscopy. Local anesthetic is used to anesthetize the surgical field. Needle entry point is determined using the intersection of the skin and the horizontal plane of the spinous process 8–13 cm lateral to the midline, depending on the level of intervention. After initial needle insertion to establish the operative approach, the needle is replaced with a guide wire. Drilling is initiated through the superior articular process (SAP) in the direction of the intervertebral disc of interest. The foramen is widened, and the ventral portion of the SAP, as well as part of the inferior articular process (IAP) are removed. After the operative window is established, sequential dilation is used to dilate the operative tunnel so that the working cannula can be

placed. Proper position of the working cannula can be confirmed with C-arm fluoroscopy (Fig. 7.1).

Throughout the procedure, a pressure regulated pump is used for rinsing the operative field with 0.9% normal saline. After the working cannula is established, discectomy and nerve root decompression is performed. Hemostasis is achieved with pressure and electrocautery, and the wound is closed. Sterile dressing is applied, and patients are instructed to follow-up postoperatively in clinic.

CERVICAL FORAMINOTOMY[2]

The patient is initially placed in a comfortable prone position under C-arm fluoroscopy. The initial skin incision is made adjacent to the cervical spinal process on the operative side at the spinal level of interest. Tubular dilators are introduced to the operative field to create a working portal window. Sequential increases in dilators are used to generate a workable operative window. The working tube is then secured over the operative lamina-facet junction (Fig. 7.2).

Foraminotomy is then performed using a high-speed drill to create a deep operative window into the stenosed spinal foramen (Fig. 7.3).

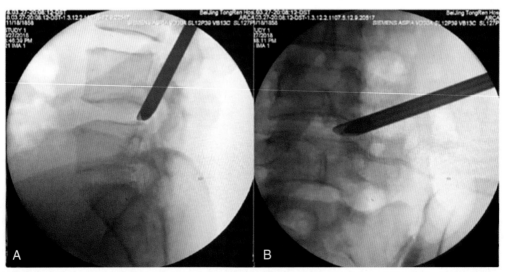

Fig. 7.1 (A) The tip of the protective cannula on the posterior rim of the upper endplate of the distal vertebrae in the lateral fluoroscopic view. (B) The tip of the protective cannula should be positioned at the medial pedicle line in the anterioposterior fluoroscopic view. (From Bao BX, Zhou JW, Yu PF, Chi C, Qiang H, Yan H. Transforaminal endoscopic discectomy and foraminoplasty for treating central lumbar stenosis. *Orthop Surg.* 2019;11:1093-1100, Figure 1.)

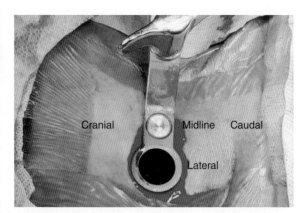

Fig. 7.2 Final operative tube placed through a 14-mm incision and secured to the table with a sterile arm. (From McAnany SJ, Qureshi SA. Minimally invasive cervical foraminotomy. *JBJS Essent Surg Tech.* 2016; 6:e23, Figure 5.)

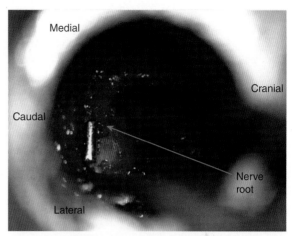

Fig. 7.4 A nerve hook used to gently retract the nerve root in a cephalad direction to inspect for any disc fragments. (From McAnany SJ, Qureshi SA. Minimally invasive cervical foraminotomy. *JBJS Essent Surg Tech.* 2016;6:e23, Figure 9.)

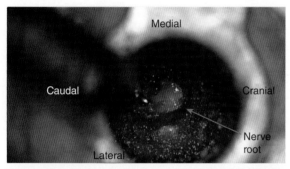

Fig. 7.3 Intraoperative photograph showing the high-speed drill being used to remove the cephalad aspect of the lamina. (From McAnany SJ, Qureshi SA. Minimally invasive cervical foraminotomy. *JBJS Essent Surg Tech.* 2016;6:e23, Figure 7.)

Foraminal decompression is then performed by using a nerve hook to retract the nerve root superiorly, after which discectomy is performed to decompress the nerve root (Fig. 7.4).

Following discectomy, hemostasis is achieved with electrocautery, and the surgical wound is closed with standard layered sutures. Following completion of foraminotomy, a sterile dressing is applied to the wound. Patients are encouraged to perform normal range of spinal motion in the postoperative period without restrictions. Follow-up is typically scheduled in clinic for 6 weeks following the procedure.

Complications

Foraminotomy is widely considered to be a safe procedure; however, as with all invasive procedures, infection, hematoma, and unintended tissue damage are possible complications. Postoperative nerve root weakness and seroma formation have also been described.[16,18] Dysesthesia is a potential complication that has been well described, and is believed to be associated with high-speed endoscopic drilling.[19,20] When it occurs, acute dysesthesia typically occurs within 1 week of the procedure and lasts for 2–4 weeks after which most patients experience a complete resolution of symptoms.[15,20] Dysesthesia is generally believed to be secondary to irritation of the exiting nerve root.[15,16]

A small number of patients may require repeat foraminotomy due to insufficient relief or rapid return of symptoms.[15] The experience and procedural skill of the interventionalist likely plays a role in this complication as recurrence of symptoms is likely due to incomplete nerve root decompression. Although uncommon, some patients require definitive management with spinal fusion to relieve symptoms of radiculopathy resistant to foraminotomy. Devastating complications of foraminotomy are exceedingly rare, but theoretically may include dural tear, meningitis, or spinal cord injury.

Conclusions

Although not widely implemented, foraminotomy is a viable intervention for the management of unilateral cervical and lumbar radiculopathy. For patients who fail to respond to medical management, and for those who are poor surgical candidates, foraminotomy may be the intervention of choice to reduce radiculopathy due to spinal foraminal stenosis. Under fluoroscopic guidance and utilizing only local anesthetic, foraminotomy is a safe procedure with minimal postoperative disruption to daily activity. With an associated low complication rate and good functional outcome, foraminotomy may become a more common practice in interventional pain clinics in the future.

REFERENCES

1. Umebayashi D, Yamamoto Y, Nakajima Y, Fukaya N, Hara M. Augmented reality visualization-guided microscopic spine surgery: transvertebral anterior cervical foraminotomy and posterior foraminotomy. *J Am Acad Orthop Surg Glob Res Rev.* 2018; 2:e008.
2. McAnany SJ, Qureshi SA. Minimally invasive cervical foraminotomy. *JBJS Essent Surg Tech.* 2016;6:e23.
3. Shu W, Zhu H, Liu R, et al. Posterior percutaneous endoscopic cervical foraminotomy and discectomy for degenerative cervical radiculopathy using intraoperative O-arm imaging. *Wideochir Inne Tech Maloinwazyjne.* 2019;14:551-559.
4. Wu PF, Li YW, Wang B, Jiang B, Tu ZM, Lv GH. Posterior cervical foraminotomy via full-endoscopic versus microendoscopic approach for radiculopathy: a systematic review and meta-analysis. *Pain Physician.* 2019;22:41-52.
5. Umebayashi D, Hara M, Nakajima Y, Nishimura Y, Wakabayashi T. Transvertebral anterior cervical foraminotomy: midterm outcomes of clinical and radiological assessments including the finite element method. *Eur Spine J.* 2013;22:2884-2890.
6. Kang KC, Lee HS, Lee JH. Cervical radiculopathy focus on characteristics and differential diagnosis. *Asian Spine J.* 2020;14: 921-930.
7. Zhang Y, Ouyang Z, Wang W. Percutaneous endoscopic cervical foraminotomy as a new treatment for cervical radiculopathy: a systematic review and meta-analysis. *Medicine (Baltimore).* 2020; 99:e22744.
8. Ruetten S, Komp M, Merk H, Godolias G. A new full-endoscopic technique for cervical posterior foraminotomy in the treatment of lateral disc herniations using 6.9-mm endoscopes: prospective 2-year results of 87 patients. *Minim Invasive Neurosurg.* 2007; 50:219-226.
9. Dodwad SJ, Dodwad SN, Prasarn ML, Savage JW, Patel AA, Hsu WK. Posterior cervical foraminotomy: indications, technique, and outcomes. *Clin Spine Surg.* 2016;29:177-185.
10. Verbiest H. A lateral approach to the cervical spine: technique and indications. *J Neurosurg.* 1968;28:191-203.
11. Song QP, Hai B, Zhao WK, et al. Full-endoscopic foraminotomy with a novel large endoscopic trephine for severe degenerative lumbar foraminal stenosis at L_5 S_1 level: an advanced surgical technique. *Orthop Surg.* 2021;13:659-668.
12. Kim HJ, Kang MS, Lee SH, et al. Feasibility of posterior cervical foraminotomy for adjacent segmental disease after anterior cervical fusion. *J Korean Neurosurg Soc.* 2020;63:767-776.
13. Ross DA, Bridges KJ. Technique of minimally invasive cervical foraminotomy. *Oper Neurosurg (Hagerstown).* 2017;13:693-701.
14. Yuchi CX, Sun G, Chen C, et al. Comparison of the biomechanical changes after percutaneous full-endoscopic anterior cervical discectomy versus posterior cervical foraminotomy at C5-C6: a finite element-based study. *World Neurosurg.* 2019; 128:e905-e911.
15. Bao BX, Zhou JW, Yu PF, Chi C, Qiang H, Yan H. Transforaminal endoscopic discectomy and foraminoplasty for treating central lumbar stenosis. *Orthop Surg.* 2019;11:1093-1100.
16. Giordan E, Billeci D, Del Verme J, Varrassi G, Coluzzi F. Endoscopic transforaminal lumbar foraminotomy: a systematic review and meta-analysis. *Pain Ther.* 2021;10:1481-1495.
17. Rubinstein SM, Pool JJ, van Tulder MW, Riphagen II, de Vet HC. A systematic review of the diagnostic accuracy of provocative tests of the neck for diagnosing cervical radiculopathy. *Eur Spine J.* 2007;16:307-319.
18. Ross DA. Complications of minimally invasive, tubular access surgery for cervical, thoracic, and lumbar surgery. *Minim Invasive Surg.* 2014;2014:451637.
19. Ahn Y, Lee SH, Park WM, Lee HY. Posterolateral percutaneous endoscopic lumbar foraminotomy for L5–S1 foraminal or lateral exit zone stenosis. Technical note. *J Neurosurg.* 2003;99:320-323.
20. Knight M, Goswami A. Management of isthmic spondylolisthesis with posterolateral endoscopic foraminal decompression. *Spine (Phila Pa 1976).* 2003;28:573-581.

Chapter 8

Laminotomy

Hamid R. Abbasi, Alaa Abd-Elsayed, and Nicholas R. Storlie

Introduction

Direct decompression of the spinal cord through laminectomy and removal of ligaments has been a traditionally common treatment for central canal stenosis.[1] During laminectomy, there is a successive removal of dorsal sources of stenosis such as the laminae, ligamentum flavum, and facet joint hypertrophy.[2] One iatrogenic consideration of laminectomy is the destabilization of the spine resulting in spondylolisthesis or hypermobility of spinal segments.[3] Additionally, traditional approaches to laminectomy may lead to ischemic damage in the surrounding musculature and poor vascularization of the bone and facet, contributing to the future progression of degeneration.[4] To improve postoperative stability of the spine while allowing for adequate decompression, less invasive surgical methods have been developed, such as facet sparing laminectomy and laminotomy.[5] In a laminotomy procedure, a caudal part of the lamina is removed unilaterally and is used as a surgical window to decompress the foramen, central canal, and lateral recesses bilaterally. This technique has been shown to have less destabilization than laminectomy in both porcine and human models and to result in comparable clinical improvements to other decompressive techniques.[6-9]

In this chapter, we describe a method of laminotomy that has been described as a tubular unilateral approach for bilateral decompression. This technique utilizes a tubular retractor as a working portal that docks onto the posterior elements of the target segment to allow for partial removal of the lamina. After a caudal part of the lamina is removed, the tubular retractor is tilted as needed for visualization. A high-speed spinal drill is used to remove the inner parts of the lamina while the

ligamentum flavum remains intact for dural protection. The tube is tilted more to perform removal of medial facet and achieve at first foraminotomy of the contralateral side. The ligamentum flavum is removed piecemeal from contralateral to ipsilateral under direct visualization of the dura, while the retractor is straightened. Finally, the ipsilateral foramen and medial facet are visualized, and the foramen is decompressed.

Indications

Indications of laminotomy for the treatment of patients with claudication and radiculopathy with:

1. Have undergone and failed an intensive nonoperative treatment that includes medication optimization, activity modification, and active physical therapy for treatment of symptoms.
2. Moderate to severe central and/or lateral recess spinal stenosis due to hypertrophy of ligaments or lamina or/and facets.

Relevant Contraindications

Laminotomy is contraindicated in any of the following scenarios:

1. Unstable spinal anatomy due to spondylolisthesis, lateral listhesis, or scoliosis.
2. Axial back pain relating to instability or degenerative disc disease is a relative contraindication.

Preoperative Considerations

Preoperatively, the patient is induced and placed in the prone position on a Jackson table. The area around the targeted levels is prepared and the draping is performed prior to surgery. Intraoperatively, 1% lidocaine with epinephrine and 0.25% Marcaine plain mixed 1:1 is injected at the skin where the incision will be made.

The side of the approach is usually the side with major symptoms or stenosis.

Postoperative Care

The patient is usually discharged on the same day with pain medication and muscle relaxants.

Complications

Complications of laminotomy include:

1. Violation of the thecal sac and nerve roots can result in iatrogenic damage to nerves and cerebrospinal fluid leak.
   a. This risk can be minimized by ensuring there is no adhesion of the dura to the ligamentum flavum and removing the ligamentum flavum after contralateral decompression.
   b. Durotomy should be repaired, if possible, directly with 4-0 Nurolon sutures. Hydrogel dural sealant (DuraSeal) may be sufficient to close the dura in smaller cases.
2. Postoperative hematoma manifesting in progressively worsening neurological symptoms.
   a. Emergent MRI should be performed to rule out hematoma, and emergency decompression may be necessary.
3. Infection of the surgical site requiring antibiotics.
4. Postoperative iatrogenic instability requiring fusion.

Laminotomy

EQUIPMENT

The method of laminotomy described is performed through a tubular retractor system (Fig. 8.1) that provides the surgeon an operative corridor. A surgical microscope is used for visualization during laminotomy (Fig. 8.2).

ANATOMY

The facet hypertrophy and ligamentum flavum/laminar hypertrophy are the targets for decompression during laminoplasty (Fig. 8.3).

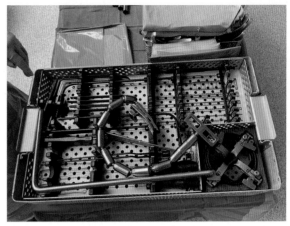

Fig. 8.1 Tray containing instruments including flexible arm, tubular retractor, dilators, and curettes.

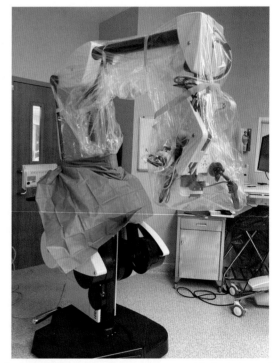

Fig. 8.2 This shows a surgical microscope used for laminotomy with proper draping.

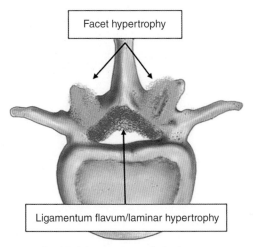

Facet hypertrophy

Ligamentum flavum/laminar hypertrophy

Fig. 8.3 Relevant anatomy for laminotomy.

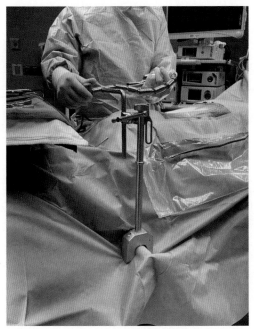

Fig. 8.4 Flex arm assembly is pictured set up to provide access to the target level.

SETUP

Patient is placed in the prone position on a Wilson frame or a flat Jackson table and appropriately draped, while the flex arm is assembled to provide access to the desired spinal level (Fig. 8.4).

EXPOSURE OF LAMINA

First, localization to the desired level is performed using fluoroscopy and a spinal needle (Fig. 8.5).

A guide wire is subsequently navigated to the inferior aspect of the targeted lamina (Fig. 8.6).

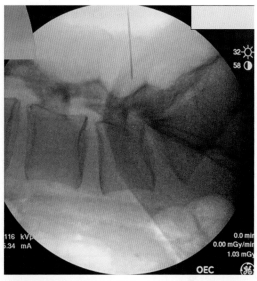

Fig. 8.5 Intraoperative fluoroscopy is used to confirm the appropriate surgical level using a spinal needle.

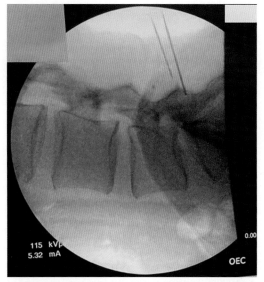

Fig. 8.6 Guidewire is placed at the inferior aspect of the targeted lamina. A 0.5- to 1-inch incision is made over the lamina unilaterally. The incision should be the size of the tubular retractor that will be placed.

After a 0.5 to 1-inch incision is made through the guide wire entry point, serial dilations are advanced down the guide wire to the inferior aspect of the lamina (Figs. 8.7–8.9).

The tubular retractor is placed over the final dilator and secured to the flexible arm (Figs. 8.10, 8.11).

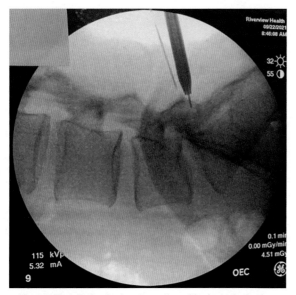

Fig. 8.7 First dilation is placed over the guidewire to the lamina.

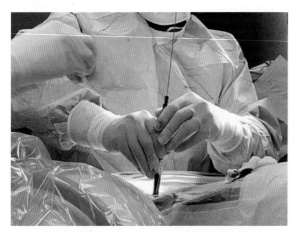

Fig. 8.8 Serial dilations are placed over the guidewire.

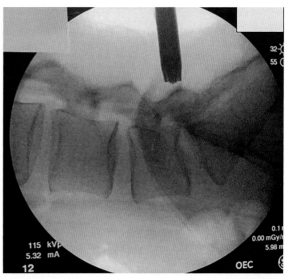

Fig. 8.9 Lateral X-ray of successive dilations to expose the lamina.

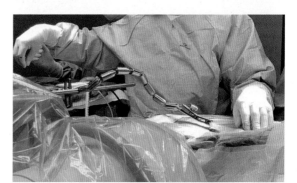

Fig. 8.10 Flexible arm is secured to the desired tubular retractor. Inner dilators are removed, establishing a surgical corridor.

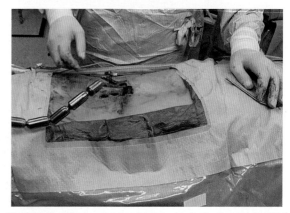

Fig. 8.11 Flexible arm securing tubular retractor in place for the third level of laminotomy.

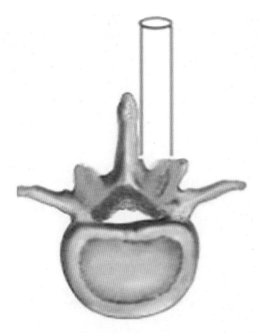

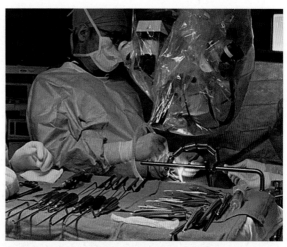

Fig. 8.13 The microscope is brought in once the tubular retractor is placed over the targeted aspect of the lamina. The inferior aspect of the lamina is removed using curved drills and bayoneted Kerrison rongeurs. The ligamentum flavum should be exposed during laminotomy but removal occurs after contralateral decompression.

Fig. 8.12 Diagram showing placement of tubular retractor during thoracolumbar laminotomy.

A diagram showing the placement of the tubular retractor anatomically is seen in Fig. 8.12.

LAMINOTOMY AND DECOMPRESSION

After the tubular retractor is appropriately placed, the microscope is brought in to visualize the lamina (Fig. 8.13).

The inferior aspect of the lamina is subsequently removed using curved drills and Kerrison rongeurs (Fig. 8.14).

The inferior lamina is removed until there is sufficient access to the ligamentum flavum and foramen (Fig. 8.15).

After an opening in the lamina has been made, the tubular retractor is tilted to access the contralateral part of the central canal through pivoting the flexible arm (Fig. 8.16).

Medial facetectomy is performed at the contralateral facet. The minimal amount of facet removal should be performed to provide decompression so that the segment will not be destabilized (Figs. 8.17–8.19).

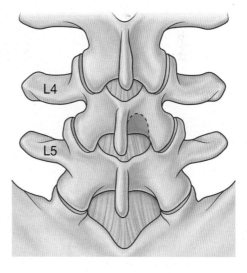

Fig. 8.14 Diagram showing location of lamina removal in lumbar laminotomy.

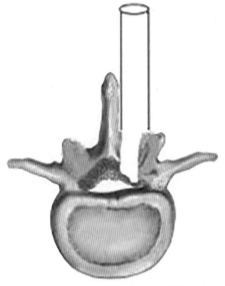

Fig. 8.15 Diagram showing initial ipsilateral partial laminectomy that provides access to the ligamentum flavum and foramen.

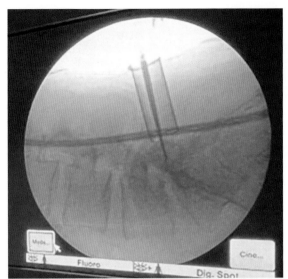

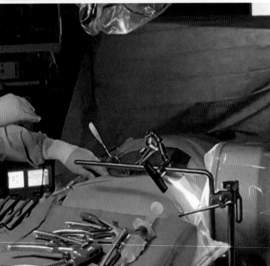

Fig. 8.17 Lateral X-ray *(left)* shows contralateral placement of curette for facetectomy as pictured on the *right*.

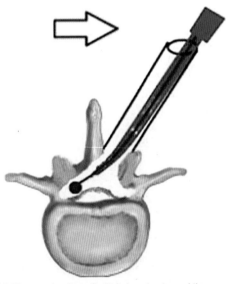

Fig. 8.16 Diagram showing a tiled tubular retractor and the removal of impinging bone of the lamina, posterior ligamentum flavum, and medial aspect of the contralateral facet/foramen. Curettes and angled drills are used to remove impinging structures. Medial facetectomy is performed at the contralateral facet. The minimal amount of facet removal should be performed to provide decompression so that the segment will not be destabilized. The arrow shoes the lateral tilting of the tubular retrator.

After contralateral foraminotomy/facetectomy is performed, the ligamentum flavum should be completely removed as the surgeon moves back toward the ipsilateral side (Fig. 8.20). The ligamentum flavum is not completely removed until after contralateral removal to keep a barrier between the surgical tools and the dura. While removing the ligamentum flavum, the largest Kerrison possible should be used in order to decrease the likelihood of a dural tear.

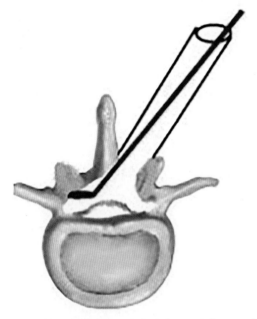

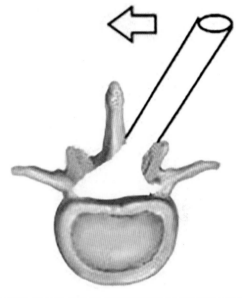

Fig. 8.18 Diagram showing curette being used for contralateral foraminotomy during lumbar laminotomy.

Fig. 8.20 Diagram showing removal of flavum following contralateral decompression.

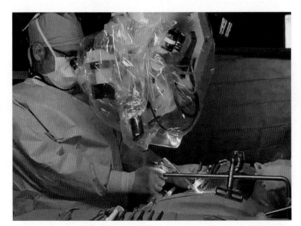

Fig. 8.19 Contralateral decompression, with tilted retractor, is performed.

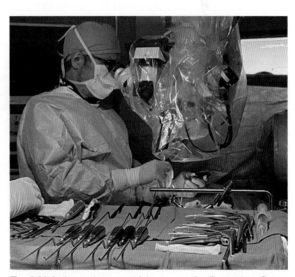

Fig. 8.21 Instruments are used to remove the ligamentum flavum completely as the retractor angle is tilted toward ipsilateral side. Removal of ligamentum flavum is confirmed when the lateral aspect of the thecal sac is visible.

The tubular retractor should be tilted stepwise as the ligamentum flavum is removed. It is important to ensure that the dura is separated from the ligamentum flavum prior to removal, which can be done with a blunt or ball-tip instrument (Fig. 8.21).

The tubular retractor angle is returned to normal as ipsilateral decompression is performed with flavum, curettes, and drills (Figs. 8.22, 8.23).

After ipsilateral decompression is complete, the tubular retractor can be removed and navigated to other levels if they are being performed (Fig. 8.24).

After laminotomy has been performed on the desired levels, the operative site is closed (Fig. 8.25).

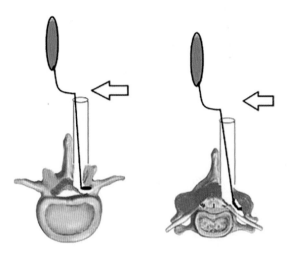

Fig. 8.22 Diagram showing removal of the flavum; curettes, drills, and Kerrisons are used to perform ipsilateral foraminotomy and medial facetectomy at a lumbar (*left*) and cervical (*right*) vertebra. The tubular retractor has been anlged back toward midline.

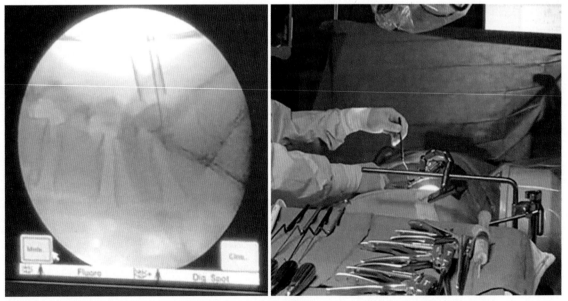

Fig. 8.23 Lateral X-ray *(left)* shows ipsilateral curette placement corresponding to the picture on the *right*.

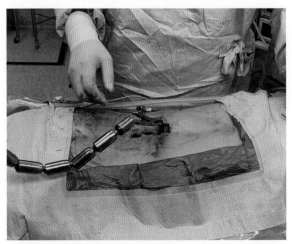

Fig. 8.24 Following laminotomy, the retractor can be removed and successive levels can be operated on if needed.

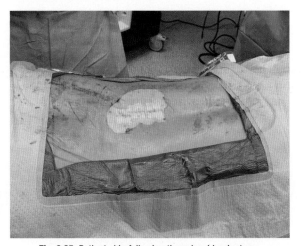

Fig. 8.25 Patient skin following three-level laminotomy.

REFERENCES

1. Airaksinen O, Herno A, Turunen V, Saari T, Suomlainen O. Surgical outcome of 438 patients treated surgically for lumbar spinal stenosis. *Spine (Phila Pa 1976)*. 1997;22(19):2278-2282.
2. Lu JJ. Cervical laminectomy: technique. *Neurosurgery*. 2007; 60(suppl 1):149-153.
3. Fox MW, Onofrio BM, Hanssen AD. Clinical outcomes and radiological instability following decompressive lumbar laminectomy for degenerative spinal stenosis: a comparison of patients undergoing concomitant arthrodesis versus decompression alone. *J Neurosurg*. 1996;85(5):793-802.
4. Rahman M, Summers LE, Richter B, Mimran RI, Jacob RP. Comparison of techniques for decompressive lumbar laminectomy: the minimally invasive versus the "classic" open approach. *Minim Invasive Neurosurg*. 2008;51(2):100-105.
5. Lee MJ, Bransford RJ, Bellabarba C, et al. The effect of bilateral laminotomy versus laminectomy on the motion and stiffness of the human lumbar spine: a biomechanical comparison. *Spine (Phila Pa 1976)*. 2010;35(19):1789-1793.
6. Tai CL, Hsieh PH, Chen WP, Chen LH, Chen WJ, Lai PL. Biomechanical comparison of lumbar spine instability between laminectomy and bilateral laminotomy for spinal stenosis syndrome - an experimental study in porcine model. *BMC Musculoskelet Disord*. 2008;9:1-9.
7. Hamasaki T, Tanaka N, Kim JH, Okada M, Ochi M, Hutton WC. Biomechanical assessment of minimally invasive decompression for lumbar spinal canal stenosis: a cadaver study. *J Spinal Disord Tech*. 2009;22(7):486-491.
8. Nerland US, Jakola AS, Solheim O, et al. Minimally invasive decompression versus open laminectomy for central stenosis of the lumbar spine: pragmatic comparative effectiveness study. *BMJ*. 2015;350:h1603.
9. Kim SK, Ryu S, Kim ES, Lee SH, Lee SC. Radiologic efficacy and patient satisfaction after minimally invasive unilateral laminotomy and bilateral decompression in patients with lumbar spinal stenosis: a retrospective analysis. *J Neurol Surgery, Part A Cent Eur Neurosurg*. 2020;81(6):475-483.

Chapter 9

Anatomic/Physiologic (Indirect) Decompression

Hamid R. Abbasi, Alaa Abd-Elsayed, and Nicholas R. Storlie

Introduction

Low back pain is a common condition affecting up to 80% of adults in the United States over the course of their lives.[1] This pain is often caused by lumbar spinal stenosis (LSS), in which nervous structures such as the spinal cord or nerve roots are compressed due to degenerative disc disease, disc herniation, or osteophytic or ligamentous hypertrophy.[2] Compression of nervous structures can also be caused by degenerative spondylolisthesis and scoliosis. These conditions can be treated through direct removal of structures that compress nerves, but the removal of disc, facet overgrowth, or elements of the posterior column can also result in iatrogenic damage to nerves and instability in some cases.[3] Another approach to nerve decompression is indirect decompression, in which the disc space of a spinal segment is increased, resulting in greater neuroforaminal space and decompressing affected nerves. Spinal interbody fusion is a type of indirect decompression in which an interbody bone graft or device is placed into the disc space following discectomy to restore disc height and expand the foramen. The placement of an interbody device loaded with biologic results in the fusion of consecutive vertebrae with an increased disc height, resulting in increase of foraminal and lateral recess space and alleviation of symptoms such as pain and radiculopathy.

Traditional lumbar fusion has been performed using an open midline technique associated with substantial blood loss, high rates of complication, and a prolonged recovery period.[4] Minimally invasive surgical (MIS) methods of interbody fusion are becoming more frequently utilized as they effectively alleviate symptoms of stenosis while reducing iatrogenic surgical morbidity.[5] MIS approaches to spinal fusion vary widely, with technologies being developed to access the disc space with anterior, lateral, and posterior approaches. In this chapter, we will discuss four different surgical methods of performing interbody fusion. Oblique lateral lumbar interbody fusion (OLLIF) is a relatively new method of lumbar interbody fusion that approaches the disc space at a 45-degree angle to the spine through the Kambin triangle, an anatomical space that permits approach without significant retraction of neural structures. Minimally invasive direct lateral interbody fusion (MIS-DLIF) approaches the disc space laterally and enters the interbody space anterior to the exiting nerve root. Minimally invasive direct thoracic interbody fusion (MIS-DTIF) is used in the thoracic region and approaches the disc space with a lateral approach. Transfacet OLLIF (TF-OLLIF), the final technique discussed, is a modification of the OLLIF that is used at the L5–S1 level in order to access a disc space through the Kambin triangle when the approach is obstructed by osteophytic changes.

Indications

OLLIF, MIS-DLIF, and TF-OLLIF are indicated for lumbar pathologies, and MIS-DTIF for thoracic pathologies, in skeletally mature patients for the treatment of low back pain and radiculopathy in patients who meet the following criteria:

1. Have undergone and failed to respond to a minimum 6 months of intensive nonoperative treatment that includes medication optimization, activity modification, and active physical therapy.

2. Severe degenerative disc disease, spondylolisthesis, discogenic stenosis, and disc rehernation are diagnosed clinically and on preoperative imaging including MRI, X-ray of the lumbar spine with flexion and extension, and computerized tomography with discogram in many cases.
3. Presence of scoliosis and other deformities, if a surgeon has sufficient experience.

Relevant Contraindications

OLLIF, MIS-DLIF, TF-OLLIF and MIS-DTIF are NOT indicated in any of the following, except in specific circumstances when other pathologies have been investigated separately and ruled out as a source of pain:
1. Any case that does not fulfill ALL of the criteria given earlier.
2. Active systemic infection or infections localized to the site of the proposed implantation are contraindications to implantation.
3. Severe osteoporosis is generally a relative contraindication for all spinal fusions because postoperative healing is impeded.
4. Any condition that significantly affects the likelihood of fusion may be a relative contraindication (e.g., cancer).
5. Comorbidities such as diabetes, osteomalacia, heavy smoking, and morbid obesity, are relative contraindications for all methods of fusion, but are smaller factors in minimally invasive fusions like those discussed in this chapter.[6]
6. These procedures can be relatively contraindicated in the following cases **depending on surgeon level of training and expertise**: bony obstruction, significant osteogenic spinal canal stenosis, large facet hypertrophy, grade II listhesis, and other gross deformities.

Preoperative Considerations

The patient should be induced followed by Foley catheter placement for longer cases. Patient is placed in the prone position on a Jackson table. Two C-arms are placed to obtain lateral and anterioposterior (AP) X-rays of the patient. The surgical site is cleaned with povidone-iodine prior to draping of the operation site.

The patient is draped, and the C-arms are draped. Skin is marked as indicated in each procedure.
Intraoperative medication includes:
1. Skin injection of 1% lidocaine with epinephrine and 0.25% Marcaine plain half/half at the injection site.
2. Lumbar epidural steroid injection (1 cc of 0.25 mg Marcaine plain with 40 cc Kenalog at the end of surgery).
3. Up to 20 cc of 0.75 mg Marcaine or Exparel in paraspinal muscles at the end of surgery.

Postoperative Care

The patient is usually discharged on the same day for smaller fusions with additional nights spent at the hospital depending on the levels fused and patient comorbidities. Patient is discharged with pain medication and muscle relaxants.

Complications

Interbody fusion is associated with several possible complications:
1. Infection of the surgical site is possible, but in our experience only occurred in 0.3% of patients.[7]
2. Nerve root irritation and damage to neural structures.
   a. A trans-Kambin approach as in our experience has a rate of nerve root irritation of 7.2%, usually involving temporary L5 numbness, decreasing to 5% after 1 year.
3. Failure to treat stenosis in 1.3% of cases, requiring patients to undergo repeat surgery.
4. Revision of posterior instrumentation is required due to screw failure occurring in a number of patients, oftentimes associated with a fall or motor vehicle accident. We found this rate to be 2% at 1-year follow-up.[8]

OLLIF: Oblique Lateral Lumbar Interbody Fusion

BACKGROUND

The oblique lateral lumbar interbody fusion (OLLIF) is a minimally invasive fusion technique that approaches the intervertebral disc space at roughly a

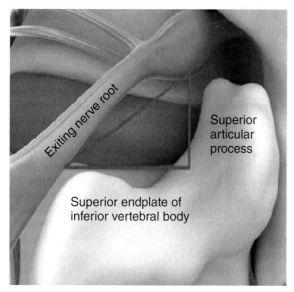

Fig. 9.1 Kambin triangle.

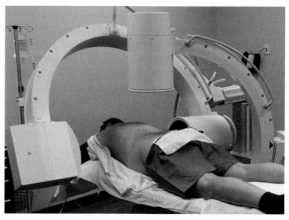

Fig. 9.2 Biplanar C-arm setup.

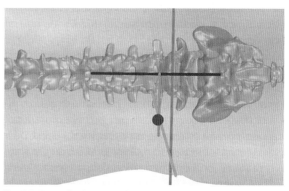

Fig. 9.3 Determination of the incision point *(purple dot)* using fluoroscopic imaging. The midline *(red line)* and target disc *(orange line)* are marked using the anterioposterior view. The lateral view is used to mark the angle of the disc on the patient's side *(green line)*.

45-degree angle from the posterior midline. OLLIF is different from other posterior approaches in that it accesses the disc space through the Kambin triangle (Fig. 9.1), an electrophysiologically silent window formed by the exiting nerve root, the superior articular process of the inferior vertebra, and the superior endplate of the inferior vertebral body. The procedure is truly minimally invasive, being performed using a Ø10-mm access portal inserted through a ~15-mm incision. The approach is guided by biplanar fluoroscopy and electrophysiological monitoring.

ROOM SETUP

The patient is placed in the prone position on a Jackson table. The table can be rotated 3–5 degrees away from the surgeon until after the cage is placed to facilitate the oblique angle of approach, but fluoroscopy must be adjusted for this (Fig. 9.2).

The endplates of the target level should be aligned in the lateral view. In the AP view, the disc should be visible, and the pedicles should be equal distances from the spinous process.

NEUROMONITORING

Electrophysiological monitoring electrodes are placed on the major muscle groups and the patient's skull to monitor somatosensory evoked potentials (SSEP) and electromyogram (EMG).

TARGETING

Determination of the incision point is performed with the use of fluoroscopic imaging. It is critical to confirm that the imaging is oriented correctly on the target level. Confirm that the AP image is properly centered over the vertebral body. This can be achieved by laying a guidewire or other radiopaque instrument on the midline to confirm that the AP image shows the pedicles are equally spaced on each side of the midline. Mark midline when fluoroscopy is centered (Fig. 9.3, red line). Next, the location of the target disc(s) should be identified, and a mark placed across the skin

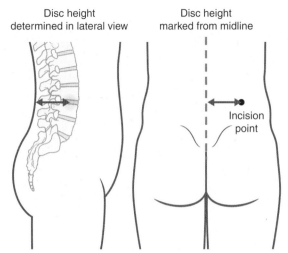

Disc height determined in lateral view

Disc height marked from midline

Incision point

Fig. 9.4 The distance from the center of the disc to the vertex of the curve of the flank (disc height) is measured, and this distance is transferred to find the distance from the midline where the incision should be made.

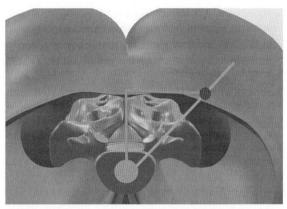

Fig. 9.5 Theoretical right triangle with the end of the hypotenuse in the center of the disc.

corresponding to the center of the disc on fluoroscopy (see Fig. 9.3, orange line).

The incision point is determined using the lateral view, with the vertebral endplates perfectly aligned. Using an opaque object to determine location, mark a line along the angle of the disc on the patient's side (see Fig. 9.3, green line). The distance from the center of the disc to the vertex of the curve of the flank is measured, and this distance is transferred to find the distance from the midline where the incision should be made (Fig. 9.4). This will create a theoretical right triangle with the end of the hypotenuse in the center of the disc (Fig. 9.5). There may be some overlap in the lengths of these lines, and the incision point should be in the approximate center of this overlap. The location of the incision is usually 10–13 cm from midline with variation based on patient disc height. The typical entry point for the OLLIF in comparison with other minimally invasive fusion approaches is displayed in Fig. 9.6.

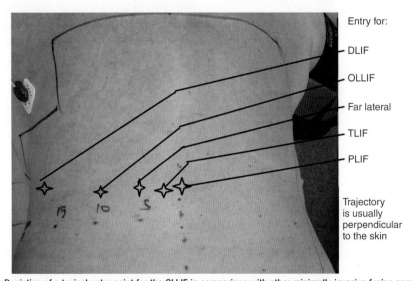

Entry for:

DLIF

OLLIF

Far lateral

TLIF

PLIF

Trajectory is usually perpendicular to the skin

Fig. 9.6 Depiction of a typical entry point for the OLLIF in comparison with other minimally invasive fusion approaches.

To confirm the incision point is in a place that will lead to the Kambin triangle without obstruction, a spinal needle may be placed to confirm the trajectory.

APPROACH

After confirming the trajectory, make a 10-mm incision in the skin and through the lumbar fascia. The electrode is stimulated at 3 mA during the approach to locate the silent window in the Kambin triangle. The neuromonitoring probe is inserted through the incision, passing through the retroperitoneal space and bluntly piercing the iliopsoas fascia (Figs. 9.7–9.9). A blunt neuromonitoring probe with sleeve is gently

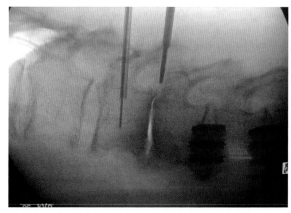

Fig. 9.9 Lateral view of the neuromonitoring probe approaching the disc space.

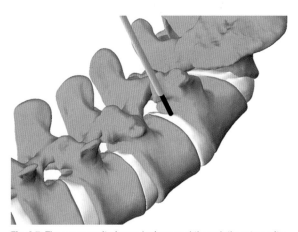

Fig. 9.7 The neuromonitoring probe is passed through the retroperitoneal space and bluntly pierces the iliopsoas fascia.

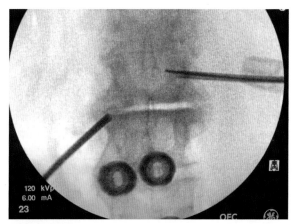

Fig. 9.10 Anterioposterior view of the neuromonitoring probe contacting the disc.

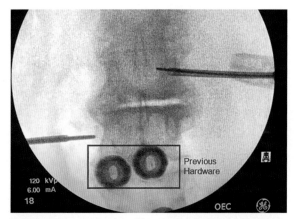

Fig. 9.8 Anterioposterior view of the neuromonitoring probe approaching the disc space.

maneuvered through the retroperitoneal space until it is positioned on the anterior aspect of the pedicle bellow, then moved along the upper side of the inferior pedicle until reaching the Kambin triangle. The electrode is stimulated at 4 mA after contacting the disc to detect possible contact with the nerve root (Figs. 9.10, 9.11). Our current data show the threshold of 3 mA is acceptable. Four of four twitches (no paralytics) is required for acceptance of the electrophysiological data. The final placement of the probe is correct when the tip is between the medial and lateral aspect of the pedicle and in the inferior section of the neural foramen (Fig. 9.12).

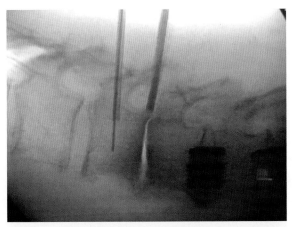

Fig. 9.11 Lateral view of the neuromonitoring probe contacting the disc.

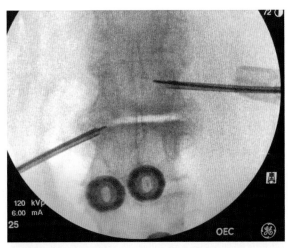

Fig. 9.13 Anterioposterior view of 18-inch guidewire being placed through the neuromonitoring probe sleeve past the midline into the disc.

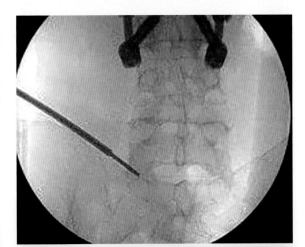

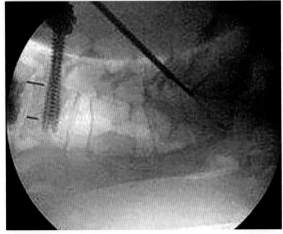

Fig. 9.12 Correct neuroprobe placement at the L5–S1 level. Anterior/Posterior XR *(top)* and lateral XR *(bottom)*.

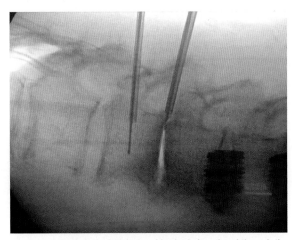

Fig. 9.14 Lateral view of 18-inch guidewire being placed through the neuromonitoring probe sleeve past the midline into the disc.

After completing the navigation to the disc, the neuromonitoring sleeve is pressed forward onto the disc and the electrode removed. An 18-inch guidewire is placed through the neuromonitoring probe sleeve past the midline into the disc (Figs. 9.13, 9.14).

Once the guidewire is correctly placed in the disc, the neuromonitoring sleeve is removed. The dilator is placed over the guidewire and fluoroscopy is used to confirm that the tip is near the center of the disc on

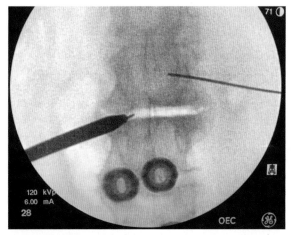

Fig. 9.15 Anterioposterior view of dilator placed over guidewire with tip near the center of the disc.

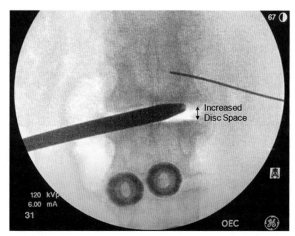

Fig. 9.17 Anterioposterior view after removal of guidewire.

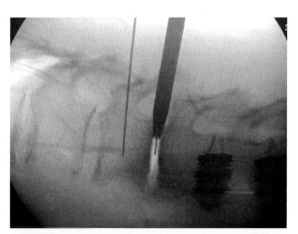

Fig. 9.16 Lateral view of dilator placed over guidewire with tip near the center of the disc.

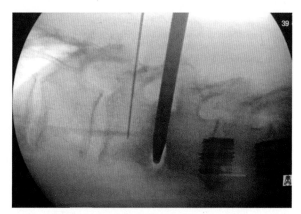

Fig. 9.18 Lateral view after removal of guidewire.

AP and lateral images (Figs. 9.15, 9.16). Insertion of the dilator should increase disc space and foraminal size, increasing the size of the silent window.

The guidewire can be removed after the dilator has entered the disc space with the correct trajectory (Figs. 9.17, 9.18).

The guidewire and the dilator handle are removed. The access portal is inserted over the dilator until the end of the portal is secured inside the disc space (Figs. 9.19, 9.20). The impact sleeve can be used to facilitate this placement. The access portal should be

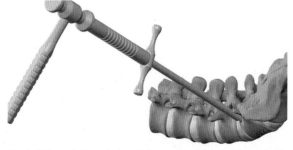

Fig. 9.19 Impact sleeve is inserted over the dilator and the mallet is used to place the access portal into the disc space.

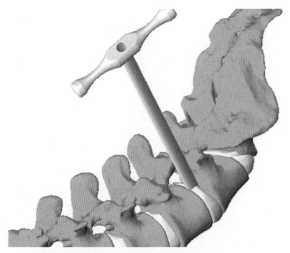

Fig. 9.20 Access portal is controlled in the disc space.

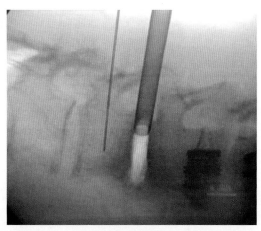

Fig. 9.22 The access portal is placed so that it is roughly 0.5 cm into the disc in the lateral view.

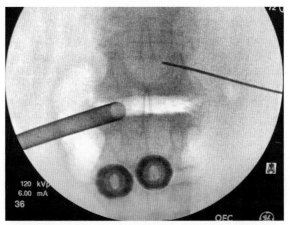

Fig. 9.21 The access portal is placed so that it is medial to the pedicle in anterioposterior view.

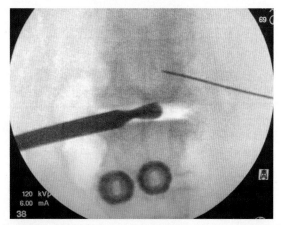

Fig. 9.23 Anterioposterior view of the 8-mm drill being introduced through the access portal.

placed so that it is medial to the pedicle in AP view (Fig. 9.21) and roughly 0.5 cm into the disc in the lateral view (Fig. 9.22).

DISCECTOMY

The 8-mm drill is introduced through the access portal to remove a segment of the nucleus pulposus and prepare a space for further discectomy instruments (Figs. 9.23, 9.24).

The distance at which the 8-mm drill protrudes past the cannula may be used to determine the

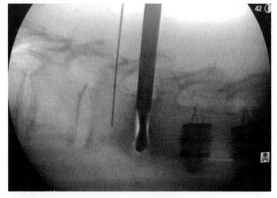

Fig. 9.24 Lateral view of the 8-mm drill being introduced through the access portal.

appropriate length of implant to be placed. Markings on the proximal shaft of the drill can be used to make this measurement.

Rotating cutter, ring curette, and long pituitary rongeur are subsequently used to debulk the nucleus of the disc and prepare the endplate (Fig. 9.25).

The flexible ring curette expands when introduced in the disc space and can be used in a fashion similar to a ring curette to scrape parallel to the endplate to ensure the endplate is free (Figs. 9.26, 9.27).

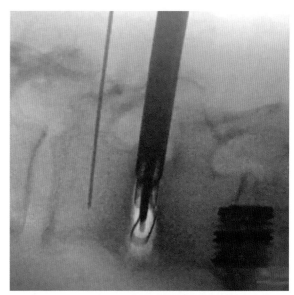

Fig. 9.27 Lateral view of flexible ring curette scraping parallel to the endplate.

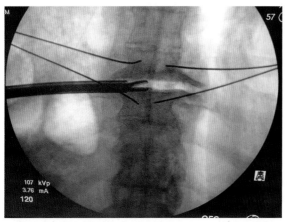

Fig. 9.25 Anteroposterior view of debulking of the nucleus and preparation of the endplate.

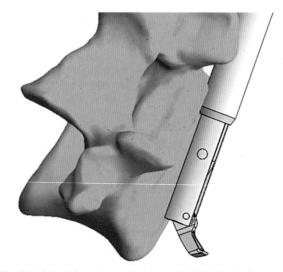

Fig. 9.28 Articulating rake curette is placed distally in the disc and used to achieve light violation of endplate.

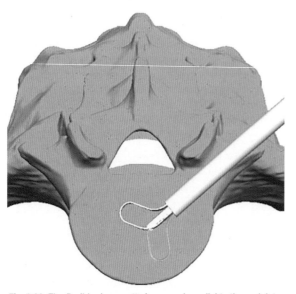

Fig. 9.26 The flexible ring curette is scraped parallel to the endplate.

The articulating rake curette functions as an angled pull cup curette with the ability to adjust in height. Place it distally in the disc and articulate the handles to push the flat rake tip against the endplate while pulling back to the cannula. Light violation of the endplates is accomplished with this instrument (Fig. 9.28).

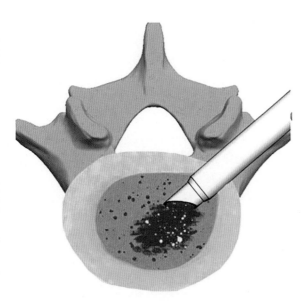

Fig. 9.29 Bone graft mixed with bone marrow aspirate is inserted into the disc space prior to insertion of the interbody cage.

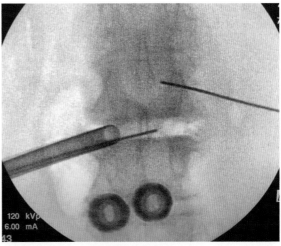

Fig. 9.30 Anterioposterior view of the guidewire placed back into the disc space as the access portal is removed.

Bone graft mixed with bone marrow aspirate obtained using a Jamshidi needle placed through the pedicle is then inserted into the disc space prior to insertion of the interbody cage (Fig. 9.29). The bone graft used in our surgeries is composed of highly purified fibrillar type I bovine collagen and resorbable 60% hydroxyapatite and 40 % tricalcium phosphate granules.

INTERBODY PLACEMENT

The guidewire is then placed back into the disc space through the access portal and the access portal is removed (Figs. 9.30, 9.31). The guidewire is placed with the blunt end facing first to reduce risk of complication.

The interbody cage is placed onto the interbody inserter and the inner part of the cage is packed with the bone graft and bone marrow aspirate mixture. The interbody is subsequently entered onto the guidewire and gently passed through, past the fascia and nerve root to the disc space (Figs. 9.32, 9.33). For easier disc entry, the cage can be rotated 90 degrees during approach and reoriented after the conical tip has entered the disc space.

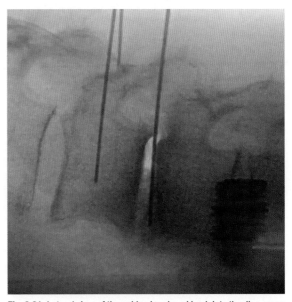

Fig. 9.31 Lateral view of the guidewire placed back into the disc space as the access portal is removed.

With mallet taps, the cage is entered into the disc until one-third of the cage is past the midline or the cage is properly oriented to fix the deformity (Figs. 9.34–9.37). Some electrophysiological activity is not unusual during cage entry. Electrophysiological

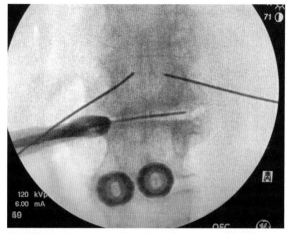

Fig. 9.32 Anterioposterior view of the interbody entering the disc space.

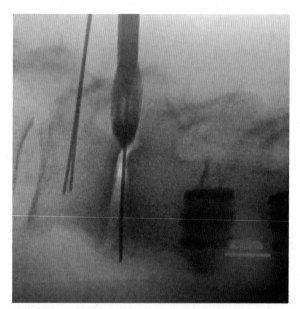

Fig. 9.33 Lateral view of the interbody entering the disc space.

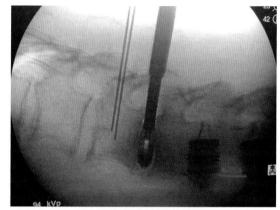

Fig. 9.34 Lateral view of the cage being positioned in the disc space.

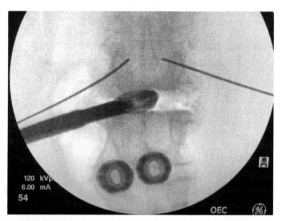

Fig. 9.35 Anterioposterior view of the cage being positioned in the disc space.

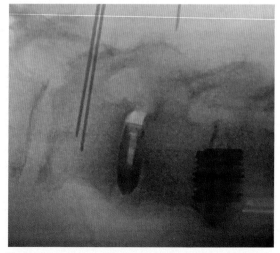

Fig. 9.36 Lateral view of the interbody cage in the proper position.

activity should subside once the cage is placed and has indirectly increased the size of the foramen.

MULTILEVEL OLLIF

Successive interbody insertion can be performed through the same incision through shifting the skin or

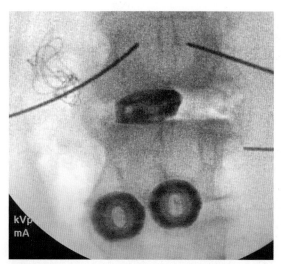

Fig. 9.37 Anterioposterior view of the interbody cage in the proper position.

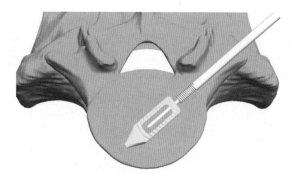

Fig. 9.39 Implant removal utilizing the guidewire and OLLIF inserter inner shaft.

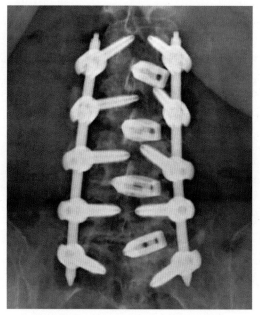

Fig. 9.38 X-ray of a completed multilevel OLLIF.

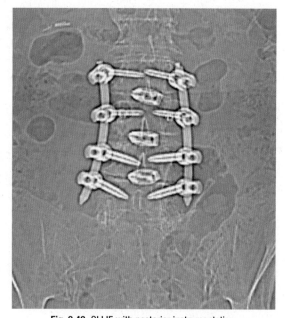

Fig. 9.40 OLLIF with posterior instrumentation.

approaching the next disc space at a slight angle. Four-level OLLIF can be seen in Fig. 9.38.

OLLIF REVISION

In the event that an implant needs to be removed after placement, follow the same surgical approach to place the dilator through the Kambin triangle. Pass a guidewire through the dilator and into the threaded aperture on the interbody device.

Remove the dilator and place the OLLIF inserter's inner shaft over the guidewire to connect to the threads of the implant. Thread the inner shaft into the implant as far as possible (Fig. 9.39).

Using a mallet, tap the inner shaft to withdraw the implant.

PEDICLE SCREW FIXATION

Insertion of the interbody is followed by percutaneous placement of pedicle screws and rods connecting all the vertebrae that are being fused (Fig. 9.40).

MIS-DLIF: Direct Lateral Lumbar Interbody Fusion

BACKGROUND

Lateral interbody fusion, which utilizes a lateral trans-psoas approach performed with the patient on their side, has become an increasingly common method of minimally invasive fusion.[9] One disadvantage of this technique as it is usually performed is the necessity to reposition the patient to prone after interbody placement for the placement of posterior screws and rods.[10] Recently, prone lateral fusion techniques have been developed in order to avoid intraoperative repositioning, but many of these techniques have few reported outcomes. MIS-DLIF is one of the earliest reported techniques of prone lateral fusion, which has been performed since 2015.[11] MIS-DLIF is a similar procedure to the OLLIF but differs in that it approaches the disc anterior to the exiting nerve root rather than through the Kambin triangle. The angle of approach is typically more lateral than the ~45 degree approach of the OLLIF, but there is variation and the procedure is a MIS-DLIF if the disc is accessed anterior to the nerve root. The MIS-DLIF is indicated for levels with high-grade listhesis or structures such as osteophytes which obstruct a trans-Kambin approach. MIS-DLIF may be preferred to OLLIF in certain cases of L5–S1 fusion, where the true OLLIF approach can be obstructed by the ala of the sacrum and iliac crest.

The MIS-DLIF has various advantages over traditional DLIF/XLIF (Figs. 9.41, 9.42). Unlike regular direct lateral procedures, MIS-DLIF does not require extensive repositioning of the patient for pedicle screw fixation, which decreases the surgical time. There is also less disruption to connective tissue and musculature due the lack of need for a larger dilation given the smaller access window. At the L4–L5 level, MIS-DLIF may be preferred due to the smaller cage size, which limits risk of injury to the lumbar plexus. Additionally, because of the variable angle of approach the L5–S1 segment is easily approachable compared with other direct lateral approach.

SETUP

Contrary to other types of lateral lumbar fusions in which the patient is placed in the lateral decubitus position, in MIS-DLIF the patient is placed in the prone position on a Jackson table (Fig. 9.43).

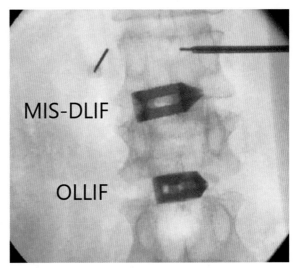

Fig. 9.41 Anterioposterior view of the cage profile for the MIS-DLIF and OLLIF approaches. The same sized cage seems longer in the anterioposterior view with MIS-DLIF

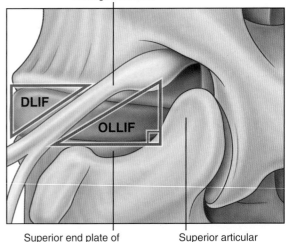

Fig. 9.42 Comparison of OLLIF and MIS-DLIF approach with respect to the exiting nerve root.

After the patient is prone, the surgical table is rotated or "helicoptered" away from the surgeon to provide better access to the more lateral angle. Biplanar fluoroscopy is used similarly to the OLLIF, but the angles must be adjusted to provide true lateral and AP views of the spine. In Fig. 9.43, the patient is seen rotated with the lateral C-arms adjusted to their anatomy.

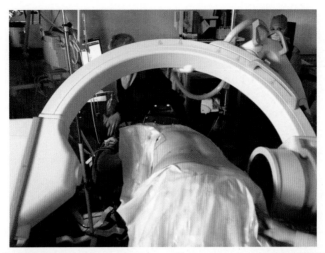

Fig. 9.43 Patient is placed in the prone position on a Jackson table for MIS-DLIF.

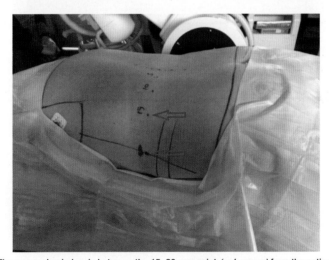

Fig. 9.44 The approach window is between the 15–20 mm point *(red arrows)* from the patient's midline.

TARGETING

The point of entry for the MIS-DLIF is more lateral than for the OLLIF. In Fig. 9.44, the approach window is shown between the 15 to 20 mm point from the patient's midline. Fig. 9.45 displays a comparison of typical DLIF and OLLIF entry points.

Like the OLLIF, the midline and targeted discs should be marked on the patient in the AP view. In the lateral view with the endplates aligned, the vertical midpoint and posterior third of the disc are projected onto the patient's skin. The incision should be placed halfway between these two points.

APPROACH

The blunt neuromonitoring probe with sleeve is entered through the incision and gently maneuvered through the abdominal muscles and the retroperitoneal space until it is positioned on the iliopsoas muscle with a trajectory to the disc space. The approach is continued with 3–4 mA stimulation to verify there is no contact with the lumbar plexus.

The approach to the disc is slightly different than in the OLLIF. In OLLIF, the tip of the electrode is medial to the border of the vertebral body (VB) in the AP

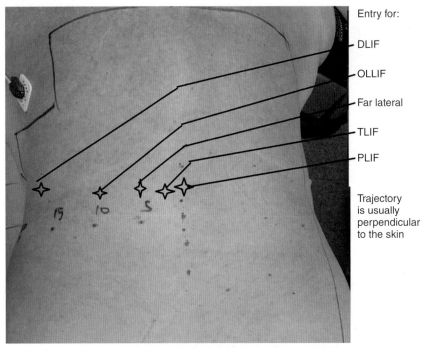

Entry for:

- DLIF
- OLLIF
- Far lateral
- TLIF
- PLIF

Trajectory is usually perpendicular to the skin

Fig. 9.45 Comparison of typical MIS-DLIF and OLLIF entry points as shown in Fig. 9.6.

view and exactly at the posterior aspect of the VB in lateral view. In MIS-DLIF, the tip of the electrode is exactly at the lateral border of the VB in the AP view, and anterior to the posterior border of the VB in the lateral view (Figs. 9.46, 9.47).

DISCECTOMY AND CAGE PLACEMENT

After the neuromonitoring probe is placed, the discectomy and cage placement proceed following the same steps as the previously described in the OLLIF procedure (Figs. 9.48–9.52).

PEDICLE SCREW FIXATION

Insertion of the interbody is followed by percutaneous placement of pedicle screws and rods connecting all the vertebrae that are being fused.

MIS-DTIF: Direct Thoracic Interbody Fusion

MIS-DLIF allows for minimally invasive placement of interbody and pedicle screws in the thoracic region (Fig. 9.53).

BACKGROUND

Minimally invasive techniques of interbody fusion such as MIS-TLIF, lateral interbody fusion, and anterior lumbar interbody fusion are difficult or impossible to apply to the thoracic spine due to anatomical considerations related to the ribcage, thoracic cavity, and pedicles.[12] Existing techniques include open surgeries with a posterior approach, lateral approach with thoracotomy, or minimally invasive endoscopic posterior approach, but these surgeries are limited by high iatrogenic tissue damage or difficult learning curves.[13,14] In this section, we describe MIS-DTIF, in which an interbody is placed through the interpleural space using biplanar fluoroscopic imaging and electrophysiological monitoring. This technique does not require thoracotomy, bone resection, or removal of aspects of a rib and is not as technically challenging as many other MIS thoracic fusion surgeries.

SETUP

The room should be set up in the same way as the OLLIF, with the biplanar fluoroscopy centered on the

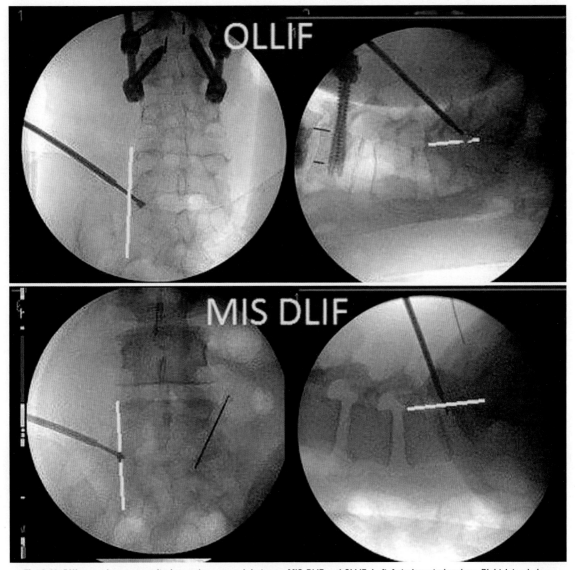

Fig. 9.46 Difference in neuromonitoring probe approach between MIS-DLIF and OLLIF. *Left,* Anterioposterior view; *Right,* lateral view.

targeted thoracic levels. Consideration needs to be given to ensure that the frame (4-post or Wilson frame) allows for proper imaging without obstruction on X-ray.

Biplanar C-arm Setup

The endplates of the target level should be aligned in the lateral view. In the AP view, the disc should be visible and the pedicles should be equal distances from the spinous process.

NEUROMONITORING

Electrophysiological monitoring electrodes is placed on the major muscle groups and the patient's skull in order to monitor SSEP and EMG.

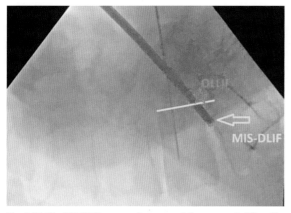

Fig. 9.47 The MIS-DLIF neuroprobe approach is more ventral than the OLLIF approach, as seen in the lateral view.

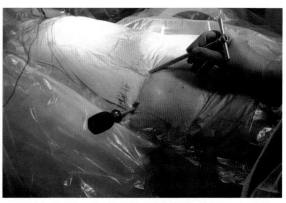

Fig. 9.48 The dilator *(black handle)* placed using MIS-DLIF approach, with the OLLIF incision point marked for comparison.

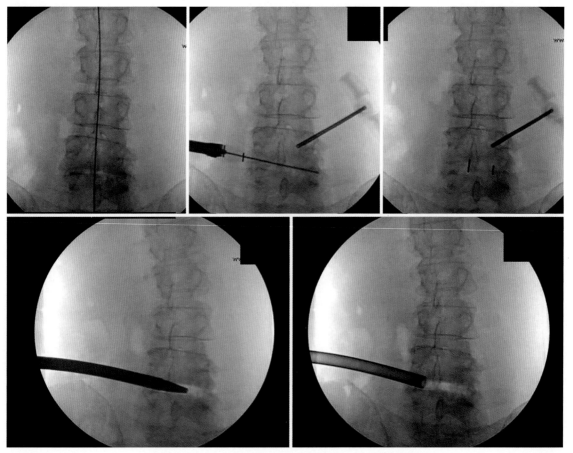

Fig. 9.49 AP view of the dilator entry and access portal placement.

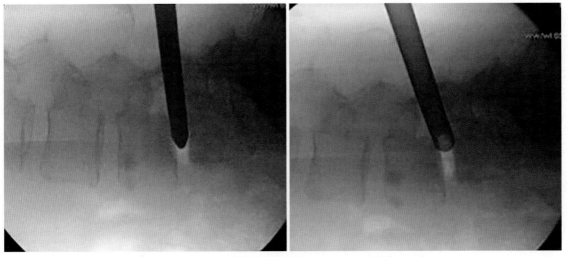

Fig. 9.50 Lateral view of the dilator entry and access portal placement.

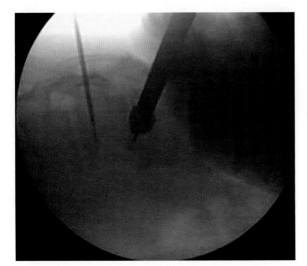

Fig. 9.51 Insertion of the cage with the MIS-DLIF approach.

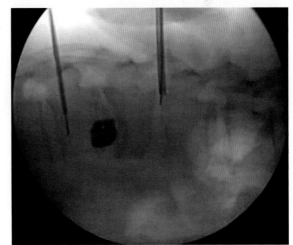

Fig. 9.52 Final cage placement utilizing an MIS-DLIF approach.

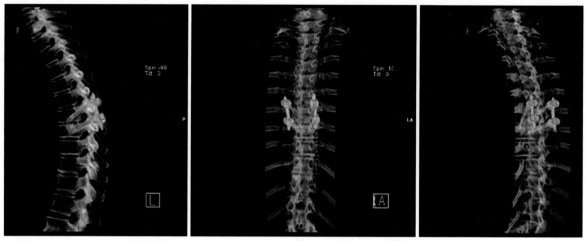

Fig. 9.53 Three-dimensional CT image of a thoracic fusion with MIS-DTIF approach.

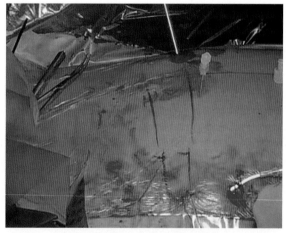

Fig. 9.54 Skin marking for MIS-DTIF.

TARGETING

Targeted discs should be marked extending laterally and a line should be marked vertically through the center of the discs and vertebral bodies (Fig. 9.54).

The incision point for MIS-DTIF is roughly at the posterior axillary line to allow for a roughly horizontal approach to the spine. The rib attaching to the inferior VB at the targeted level is identified and an incision is placed just above this rib on the posterior axillary line to protect costal neurovascular structures.

APPROACH

An ~0.5 cm opening in the intercostal ligament is performed with a Kelly clamp, which should be undersized to achieve sealing of the pleural space. A blunt cannulated 8-mm dilator probe is inserted into the pleural space and the surgeon should make tactile and fluoroscopic confirmation of contact with the inferior rib (Figs. 9.55, 9.56).

Following contact with the rib, the dilator should be advanced along the course of the rib, keeping constant contact with the rib until reaching the rib head and the disc space. The guidance for this approach is both tactile and fluoroscopic (Figs. 9.57, 9.58).

Correct placement of the dilator is confirmed with biplanar fluoroscopy, as free hand placement has been shown to be unreliable (Fig. 9.59).

After the dilator has been guided to the entrance of the disc and firmly positioned, a sharp tipped guidewire is introduced into the cannulated dilator and into the disc space. The dilator is tapped into the disc space using a mallet and the guidewire is removed

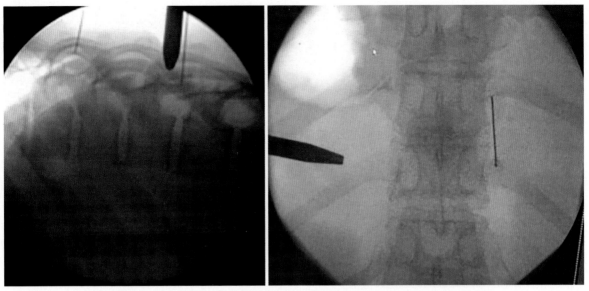

Fig. 9.55 Lateral view *(left)* and anterioposterior view *(right)* of dilator approaching the targeted rib.

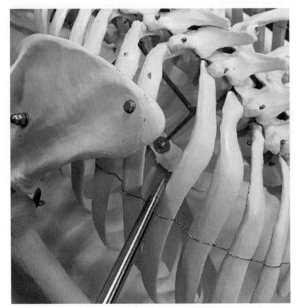

Fig. 9.56 Demonstration of the dilator making contact with the inferior rib.

after the dilator is positioned in the disc. A working channel is inserted over the dilator to the edge of the disc space and the dilator can be removed (Fig. 9.60).

DISCECTOMY AND CAGE PLACEMENT

Discectomy is performed in the same manner as the OLLIF (Fig. 9.61).

Bone graft is inserted following discectomy and the guidewire is inserted back to the disc space. The access portal is removed, and the cage is inserted to the disc space on the guidewire (Fig. 9.62). The cage is typically inserted with a mallet until one-third of the cage is past the midline.

Following cage insertion, the pleural space is sutured in two layers.

PEDICLE SCREW FIXATION

Insertion of the interbody is followed by percutaneous placement of pedicle screws and rods connecting all the vertebrae that are being fused.

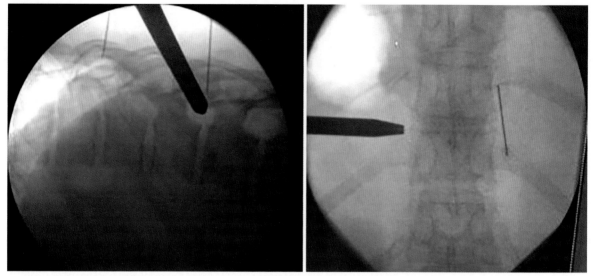

Fig. 9.57 Lateral *(left)* and anterioposterior *(right)* views of the dilator approaching the head of the rib and disc space.

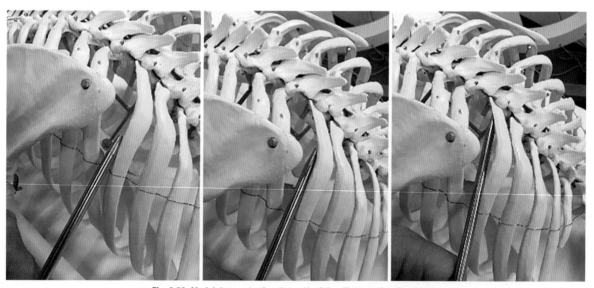

Fig. 9.58 Model demonstrating the path of the dilator to the disc space.

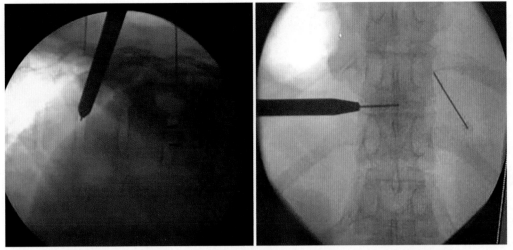

Fig. 9.59 Lateral *(left)* and anterioposterior *(right)* view of the dilator centered on the disc space.

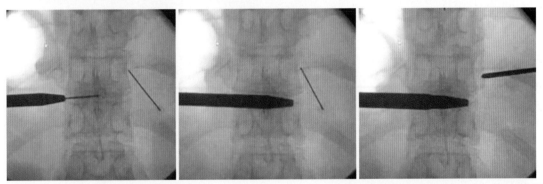

Fig. 9.60 AP view of guidewire placement *(left)*, correct dilator positioning *(middle)*, and insertion of access portal over the dilator *(right)*.

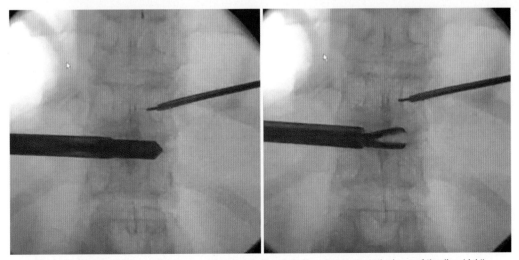

Fig. 9.61 AP view of drill used to clear space in disc *(left)* and pituitary rongeur to grab pieces of the disc *(right)*.

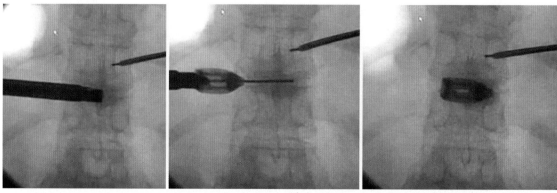

Fig. 9.62 AP view of bone graft inserted *(left)*, cage approaching disc space on the guidewire *(middle)*, and final cage placement *(right)*.

Transfacet OLLIF

BACKGROUND

One of the limitations of OLLIF is the possible obstruction of the Kambin triangle at the L5–S1 level by prominent sacral ala or osteophytic growth surrounding a pathological facet joint. In these cases, it may be difficult to pass a neuromonitoring probe into the disc space and place an interbody through the compressed space. TF-OLLIF was developed as a way to access the disc space with an OLLIF approach in cases where facet hypertrophy previously prevented OLLIF. Typically, TF-OLLIF will be attempted in the case that an electrophysiologically silent approach cannot be performed in typical OLLIF fashion. A drill is used to remove facet hypertrophy and allow access to the disc.

ROOM SETUP

Generally identical to OLLIF: Patient is placed in the prone position on a Jackson table (Fig. 9.63). The table can be rotated 3–5 degrees away from the surgeon until after the cage is placed to facilitate the oblique angle of approach, but fluoroscopy must be adjusted for this.

The endplates of the target level should be aligned in the lateral view. In the AP view, the disc should be visible and the pedicles should be equal distances from the spinous process.

Neuromonitoring

Electrophysiological monitoring is placed on the major muscle groups and the patient's skull in order to monitor SSEP and EMG.

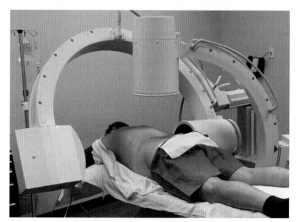

Fig. 9.63 Biplanar C-arm setup for TF-OLLIF.

TARGETING

Targeting for TF-OLLIF is the same as OLLIF.

APPROACH

Approach for the TF-OLLIF starts with a neuromonitoring probe being advanced toward the disc space at the same 45 degree angle used in OLLIF. After the determination to use the TF-OLLIF technique has been made, the probe should be docked on the lateral aspect of facet that would typically allow for an OLLIF approach with a trajectory that would take the probe to the center of the disc (Fig. 9.64).

A sharp guidewire is docked and gently malleted onto the bone. A cannulated dilator is inserted onto the guidewire down to the bone (Fig. 9.65).

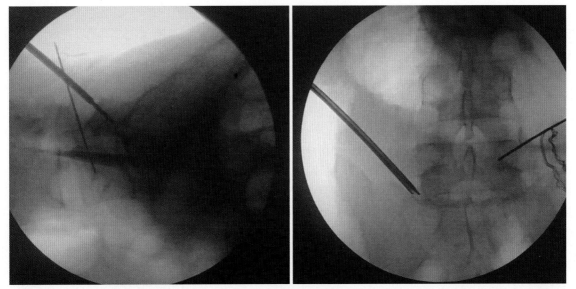

Fig. 9.64 Lateral view *(left)* and anteriorposterior view *(right)* of the probe docked on bone allowing a good trajectory to the disc space.

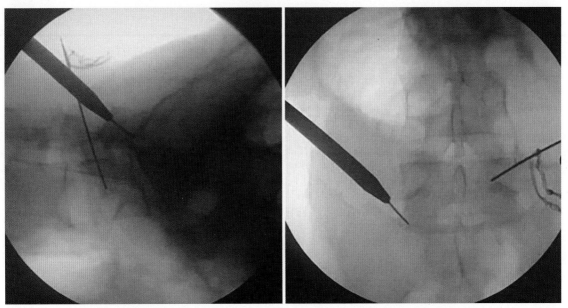

Fig. 9.65 Lateral view *(left)* and anteriorposterior view *(right)* of the dilator inserted down to the facet.

The access portal should be inserted over the dilator and inserted until contact with the facet (Fig. 9.66). The guidewire can be removed at this point and the trajectory of the dilator/access portal can be adjusted.

The dilator can be removed after the access portal is inserted and a drill is inserted through the access portal (Fig. 9.67). The drill is used to remove the bone obstructing a pathway to the disc, while the access portal advances following removal of bone (Fig. 9.68). Continued stimulation between 10–12 mA is performed during the approach; a threshold of 8 mA is acceptable.

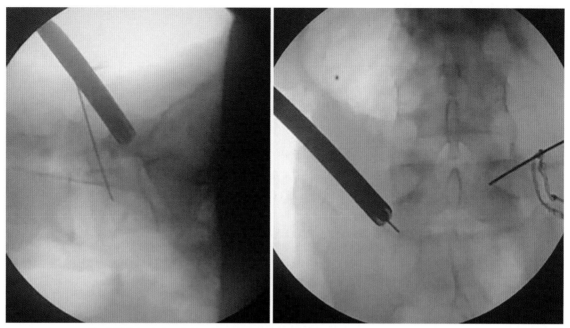

Fig. 9.66 Lateral view *(left)* and anterioposterior view *(right)* of the dilator and guidewire inserted.

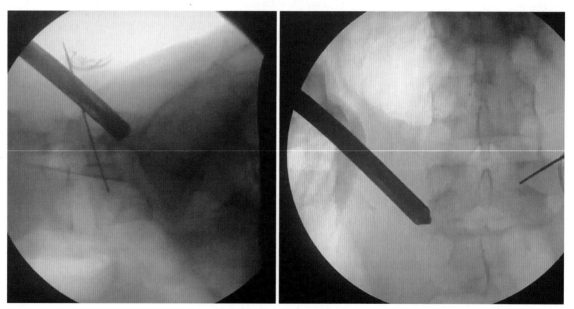

Fig. 9.67 Lateral view *(left)* and anterioposterior view *(right)* of the drill being advanced.

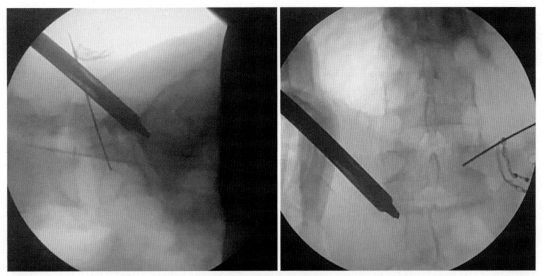

Fig. 9.68 Lateral view *(left)* and anterioposterior view *(right)* of the drill advanced further to the disc.

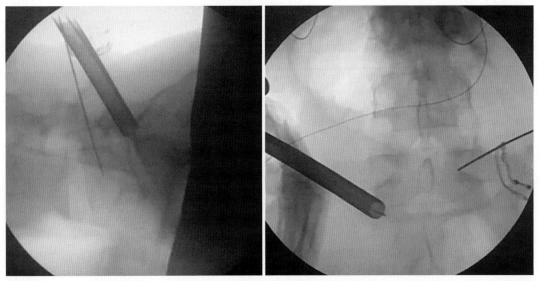

Fig. 9.69 Lateral view *(left)* and anterioposterior view *(right)* of the guidewire inserted through the access portal to the edge of the disc space.

After the bone obstructing access to the disc has been removed, the guidewire is inserted through the access portal blunt end first into the disc space (Fig. 9.69).

The guidewire is removed from the access portal and the dilator is inserted to open the disc space and allow entry of the access portal (Fig. 9.70).

DISCECTOMY AND CAGE PLACEMENT

Discectomy is performed in a similar manner to OL-LIF (Figs. 9.71, 9.72).

PEDICLE SCREW FIXATION

Insertion of the interbody is followed by percutaneous placement of pedicle screws and rods connecting all the vertebrae that are being fused.

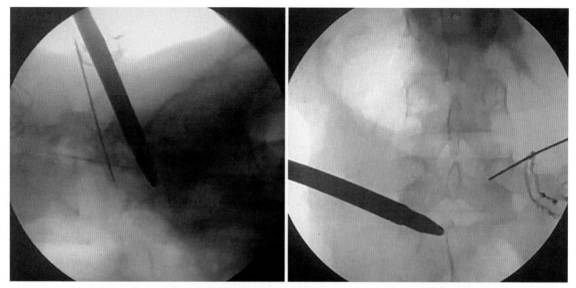

Fig. 9.70 Lateral view *(left)* and anterioposterior view *(right)* of the dilator being inserted into the disc space.

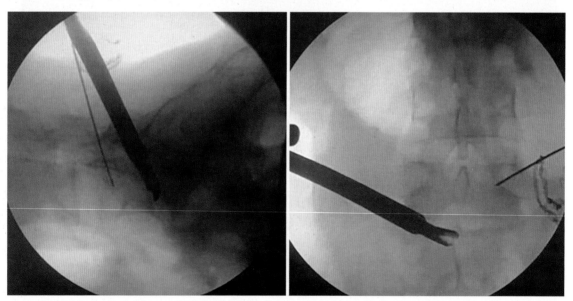

Fig. 9.71 X-ray of articulating curette *(left)* and pituitary rongeur *(right)* being used in the disc space to perform discectomy.

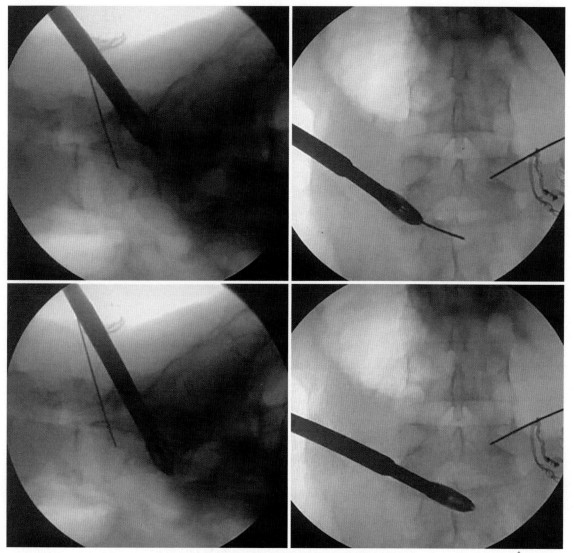

Fig. 9.72 X-ray of cage being placed with a transfacet approach.

REFERENCES

1. Urits I, Burshtein A, Sharma M, et al. Low back pain, a comprehensive review: pathophysiology, diagnosis, and treatment. *Curr Pain Headache Rep.* 2019;23(3):1-10.
2. Lurie J, Tomkins-Lane C. Management of lumbar spinal stenosis. *BMJ.* 2016;352:h6234.
3. Yoshihara H. Indirect decompression in spinal surgery. *J Clin Neurosci.* 2017;44:63-68.
4. Patel AA, Zfass-Mendez M, Lebwohl NH, et al. Minimally invasive versus open lumbar fusion: a comparison of blood loss, surgical complications, and hospital course. *Iowa Orthop J.* 2015;35:130-134.
5. Goldstein CL, Macwan K, Sundararajan K, Rampersaud YR. Comparative outcomes of minimally invasive surgery for posterior lumbar fusion: a systematic review. *Clin Orthop Relat Res.* 2014;472(6):1727-1737.
6. Park P, Upadhyaya C, Garton HJL, Foley KT. The impact of minimally invasive spine surgery on perioperative complications in overweight or obese patients. *Neurosurgery.* 2008;62(3):693-698.
7. O'Toole JE, Eichholz KM, Fessler RG. Surgical site infection rates after minimally invasive spinal surgery: clinical article. *J Neurosurg Spine.* 2009;11(4):471-476.
8. Abbasi A, Khaghany K, Orandi V, Abbasi H. Clinical and radiological outcomes of oblique lateral lumbar interbody fusion. *Cureus.* 2019;11(2):e4029.

9. Uribe JS, Deukmedjian AR. Visceral, vascular, and wound complications following over 13,000 lateral interbody fusions: a survey study and literature review. *Eur Spine J.* 2015;24:386-396.

10. Godzik J, Ohiorhenuan IE, Xu DS, et al. Single-position prone lateral approach: cadaveric feasibility study and early clinical experience. *Neurosurg Focus.* 2020;49(3):1-8.

11. Abbasi H, Abbasi A. Minimally invasive direct lateral interbody fusion (MIS-DLIF): proof of concept and perioperative results. *Cureus.* 2017;9(1):1-9.

12. Smith JS, Ogden AT, Fessler RG. Minimally invasive posterior thoracic fusion. *Neurosurg Focus.* 2008;25(2):1-9.

13. Lin B, Shi JS, Zhang HS, Xue C, Zhang B, Guo ZM. Subscapularis transthoracic versus posterolateral approaches in the surgical management of upper thoracic tuberculosis a prospective, randomized controlled study. *Med (United States).* 2015;94(47):e1900.

14. Yue B, Chen B, Zou YW, et al. Thoracic intervertebral disc calcification and herniation in adults: a report of two cases. *Eur Spine J.* 2016;25:118-123.

Chapter 10

Measuring Outcomes in Spinal Decompression

Alyson M. Engle and Merna Naji

Introduction

In patients with spinal disorders that warrant spinal decompression, the goal of intervention is to enhance function and reduce pain. In the past, outcomes were commonly assessed based on the results of imaging as well as the interventionalist's subjective views; however, studies have shown that these frequently do not correlate with patient satisfaction.[1,2] In one study, Schwartz et al. reported an astonishing 24% mismatch in physician–patient perceived outcomes after spinal surgery.[3] Patient-reported outcome measures (PROM) were created out of necessity to derive quantitative data from a patient's perceived health. More recently, several questionnaires have been developed and validated to evaluate the severity of a condition and response to intervention. Such data aim to help providers develop a treatment plan and follow the patient to determine treatment efficacy. PROMs have a place not only in the clinical setting but also in research to help advance the field of interventional spine care (Table 10.1).

Indications for Use of Each Instrument

Many clinicians utilize the familiar numeric pain rating system (NRS) and/or the visual analog scale (VAS) to quickly assess pain intensity. The NRS is an 11-point numerical rating scale used to measure pain intensity. The patient is asked to choose a number between 0 and 10 that best represents how much pain they are feeling that day. Zero generally represents "no pain at all" whereas ten represents "the worst possible pain." Alternatively, the VAS has many different versions. Examples of the most commonly

used ones include a VAS of faces that asks patients to identify a face that best represents their perception of their pain. Alternatively, a metric VAS is one in which the patient marks a point on a 100-mm horizontal line that represents zero pain on one end and the highest amount of pain on the other. One then measures the distance from the beginning of the line to the marked point and the pain intensity is computed in millimeters. Although widely used and validated to show high correlation with other pain assessment tools,[14] the NRS and VAS have been criticized for being unable to capture the complex, multifactorial, and functional burden of pain. As a result, more sophisticated patient-reported outcome (PRO) instruments have been developed over time. This chapter will focus on instruments for measuring outcomes in spinal decompression.

The most widely used measurement tool for assessing health-related quality of life is the Medical Outcomes Study Short Form questionnaire (SF-36). The SF-36 was derived from the Medical Outcomes Study, a multi-year study performed to elucidate variations in patient outcomes and to develop functional tools for monitoring patient outcomes and their determinants.[6] The survey is composed of 36 questions that are organized into eight domains. The questions focus on the degree of limitation caused by the patient's health on numerous activities. The results are expressed on a scale ranging from 0 to 100 with higher values representing better function. It is easy to see why it is a widely used instrument, as it is a generic tool that has been validated for a broad spectrum of spine pathologies and procedures including discectomy,[15] decompressive laminectomy,[16] and fusion.[17] The SF-12 and SF-6 are shortened versions of the SF-36, created to reduce the burden of response. There are data showing

TABLE 10.1 Outcome Measurement Instruments

Instrument	Measurement	Scoring Description	MCID[a]
Numerical Pain Rating Scale (NRS)	Pain intensity	Evaluates pain intensity. Patients choose a number between 0 and 10 that best represents how much pain they are feeling that day. 0 represents "no pain at all" whereas 10 represents "the worst possible pain."	1–2[4]
Visual Analog Scale (VAS)	Pain intensity	Evaluates pain intensity. Examples: 1) VAS of cups which relates the amount of liquid inside a glass to the intensity of the pain perceived by the patient 2) VAS of faces in which the patient picks the illustrated emotion that best represents their level of pain 3) Metric VAS in which the patient marks a spot on a 100 mm horizontal line that represents zero pain on one end and the most amount of pain on the other. The pain intensity is computed in millimeters.	30 mm (Metric VAS)[5]
Short Form- 36 (SF-36)	General health and debility status	Assesses health-related quality of life.[15] Derived from the Medical Outcomes Study[6] and is composed of 36 questions that are organized into 8 domains. The questions focus on the degree of limitation caused by the patient's health on numerous activities. The results are expressed on a scale ranging from 0 to 100 with higher values representing better function. Truncated versions include the SF-6 and SF-12.[7]	4.9[4]
The RAND 36-Item Health Survey 1.0 (RAND-36)	General health and debility status	Assess health-related quality of life. The RAND-36 and SF-36 include the same set of eight domains that were developed in the Medical Outcomes Study.[6] The scoring of the domains yields equivalent results for six out of the eight subscales.[8] Designed to reduce the burden of respondents.	—
Patient-Reported Outcomes Measurement Information System (PROMIS)	General health and debility status	Measure pain intensity using a 0 through 10 numeric rating system over seven health domains. Scores are standardized against US normative population data.[9]	—
Oswestry Disability Index (ODI)	Back disability	Evaluate the limitations of back pain on different daily activities of living. There are 10 questions with each scored from 0 to 5, with 5 representing the most significant disability. The maximum score is 50 and the patient's total can be multiplied by 2 to produce a percentage score.	12.8[4]
Roland-Morris Disability Questionnaire (RMDQ)	Back disability	Assess the impact of lower back pain on daily life and work activities. Consists of 24 statements and the results vary from 0 (no impairment) to 24 (severe impairment).	3–5[10]
Quebec Back Pain Disability Scale (QBPDS)	Back disability	Measure the degree of disability caused by back pain. It is composed of 20 activities and asks patients to rate their perceived amount of difficulty in performing each activity from 0 (not difficult at all) to 5 (unable to do). The responses are summed for a total score between 0 and 100 with a higher score representing a greater degree of disability.	—
Zurich Claudication Questionnaire (ZCQ)	Back disability	Measure treatment outcomes in patients with lumbar spinal stenosis. There are 12 questions for all patients and an additional 6 for patients who have undergone spinal intervention. The score is expressed as a percentage with a higher score representing a greater degree of disability.	—

TABLE 10.1 Outcome Measurement Instruments—cont'd			
Instrument	**Measurement**	**Scoring Description**	**MCID[a]**
Neck Disability Index (NDI)	Neck disability	Assess self-rated disability in patients with neck pain.[11] It is scored similarly to the ODI in that there are 10 questions with each one scored from 0 to 5 with 5 representing the most significant disability. The maximum score is 50 and the patient's total can be multiplied by 2 to produce a percentage score.	7.5[12]
Beck Depression Inventory (BDI)	Psychological status	Evaluate degree of depression. Consists of 21 questions with scores ranging from 0 to 3. Scores range from 0 to 63. Scores of 0 to 13 indicate no depression or minimal symptoms, scores of 14 to 19 indicate mild depression, scores of 20 to 28 indicate moderate depression, and scores of 29 to 63 indicate severe depression.	17.5%–32%[13]

[a]MCID is the Minimal Clinically Important Difference, which represents the smallest change that a patient would rate as meaningful. Outcome measurement instruments are free to use except for the PROMIS and ODI tools.

PROMIS and ODI are copyright and free to use only for nonfunded academic research and individual clinical practice. Other uses are subject to a fee.

that the SF-12 is a valid alternative to the SF-36 for preoperative and postoperative assessments of health status in patients with lumbar surgical disorders undergoing decompression surgery for a predominant symptom of radiating leg pain.[18] When compared with the SF-36, the SF-12 and SF-6 scores were similar but almost always had larger standard errors.[7] The RAND-36 (distributed by RAND corporation) includes the same set of eight domains that were developed in the SF-36 and Medical Outcomes Study. The scoring of the domains yields equivalent results for six out of eight of the domains; however, scoring differences exist for the pain and general health subscales. The detailed differences in scoring are summarized by Hays, Sherbourne, and Mazel.[8]

Another generic tool for measuring health-related quality of life across a variety of chronic diseases is the Patient-Reported Outcomes Measurement Information System (PROMIS). The PROMIS-29 profile assesses pain intensity using a 0 through 10 numeric rating system over seven health domains (physical function, fatigue, pain interference, depressive symptoms, anxiety, ability to participate in social roles and activities, and sleep disturbance). Scores are standardized against United States normative population data. PROMIS has been compared with the SF-12 and Neck Disability Index (NDI) and is validated for patients treated

surgically for degenerative cervical spine disorders.[19] It has additionally been compared with the Oswestry Disability Index (ODI) and Zurich Claudication Questionnaire (ZCQ) and is additionally validated for patients treated surgically for lumbar spinal stenosis.[20]

Unlike the generic tools discussed earlier, there are numerous disease-specific outcome measures unique to spine that link functional impairment reported by the patient to spine pathology. The ODI is the scale most commonly used to assess disability in low back pain and lumbar spine pathologies. There are 10 questions, each scored from 0 to 5, with 5 representing the most significant disability. The maximum score is 50 and can be multiplied by 2 to produce a percentage score. Scores between 0%–20% indicate minimal disability; 20%–40% indicate moderate disability; 40%–60% indicate severe disability; 60%–80% indicate crippling back pain; and 80%–100% describe patients who are bed-bound or exaggerating their symptoms. Generally, patients who score in the mild and moderate disability range can be treated with conservative measures, which include improved posture as well as general health and physical activity advice. Patients who score in the severe and crippling back pain ranges require further investigation and likely intervention. It is recommended that the ODI be administered to the patient to obtain an original baseline and then every two weeks after the intervention to measure progress. The ODI is considered the gold standard outcome tool for assessing function in activities of daily living in low back pain. It has been repeatedly validated in patients with lumbar spine pathologies.

Other instruments that assess disability due to lower back disorders include the Roland-Morris Disability Questionnaire (RMDQ) and Quebec Back Pain Disability Scale (QBPDS). The RMDQ is more appropriate for the assessment of patients with mild-moderate disabilities whereas the ODI may be more valid at measuring higher disability levels.[21] The RMDQ consists of 24 statements that assess the impact of low back pain in daily life and work activities. The results vary from 0 (no impairment) to 24 (severe impairment). There are over 50 translations and adaptations available for application. Alternatively, the QBPDS is a measure that was described by Kopec and colleagues in 1995 to measure disability caused by back pain. The scale is composed of 20 activities and asks patients to rate their perceived amount of difficulty in performing each activity from 0 (not difficult at all) to 5 (unable to do). The responses are summed for a total score between 0 and 100 with a higher score representing a greater degree of disability.

The first tool designed to assess disability in patients with neck pain is the NDI.[12] Similar to the ODI, the NDI has 10 questions with each one scored from 0 to 5 with 5 representing the most significant disability. The maximum score is 50 and can be multiplied by two to produce a percentage score. It has been validated for those undergoing cervical fusion for degenerative spine disorders.[22]

Alternatively, the ZCQ is a tool designed for patients with lumbar spinal stenosis. There are 12 questions for all patients and an additional 6 for patients who have undergone intervention. The score is expressed as a percentage, with a higher score representing a greater degree of disability.

Perioperative Considerations

Perioperative psychological evaluation is important in the preoperative and postoperative period. The presence of depression and anxiety in the preoperative period is associated with increased failure rates after surgical decompression for degenerative diseases of the spine.[23,24] The most widely used psychological assessment tool is the Beck Depression Inventory (BDI). The BDI consists of 21 questions with scores ranging from 0 to 3. The instrument assesses sadness, pessimism, sense of failure, feelings of guilt, self-dislike, suicidal thoughts, weight loss, work inhibition, sleep disturbances, fatigability, and loss of libido. Total scores range from 0 to 63. Scores of 0 to 13 indicate no depression or minimal symptoms, scores of 14 to 19 indicate mild depression, scores of 20 to 28 indicate moderate depression, and scores of 29 to 63 indicate severe depression.

General Considerations

Successful PRO instruments are reliable, validated, yield appropriate responsiveness, decrease administrative burden and cost, and have language adaptations. The aforementioned PROs are among the most common in use today and have been validated for a variety of spine disorders. Some instruments have truncated versions, such as the SF-12, that were created to reduce the burden of response. Others, such as PROMIS, have developed computer-adaptive testing in which the questions are tailored to each person under evaluation. Many of the above PROs are available in numerous languages as well as cultural versions, such as the ODI, which has over 31 adaptations.[25]

Another attribute for a successful PRO is interpretability. When assessing the clinical utility of spine surgery, one must determine the amount of subjective change that is most important to the patient. This is best expressed as the Minimal Clinically Important Difference (MCID), which is the smallest change that a patient would rate as meaningful. The two most widely used approaches to determine the MCID are anchor-based and distribution-based methods. We will avoid getting into the heavy details of statistics in this chapter, however it is important to note that limitations exist in the determination of the MCID. Schwartz et al. provide an exemplary paraphrase of such limitations. They note that "each method [of determining MCID] produces an MCID value different from the other methods.

MCID definitions do not take into account the cost of treatment to the patient, and the change in PRO scores depends on the patient's initial baseline status".[26] Some studies report the percentage of "responders" to a certain intervention. A responder is any patient who reaches the MCID threshold, and although not perfect, it serves as an important data point for clinicians in anticipating what portion of patients can be expected to benefit from an intervention. A range of the most agreed-upon MCIDs are expressed in the table above.

In general, there are many validated PRO instruments available that measure different clinical and functional outcomes, and it is essential for spine care providers to have good command and use of the PRO instruments.

REFERENCES

1. Goni VG, Hampannavar A, Gopinathan NR, et al. Comparison of the Oswestry Disability Index and magnetic resonance imaging findings in lumbar canal stenosis: an observational study. *Asian Spine J.* 2014;8(1):44-50.
2. Weber C, Giannadakis C, Rao V, et al. Is there an association between radiological severity of lumbar spinal stenosis and disability, pain, or surgical outcome? A multicenter observational study. *Spine (Phila Pa 1976).* 2016;41(2):E78-E83.
3. Schwartz CE, Armon A, Finkelstein JA. When patients and surgeons disagree about surgical outcome: investigating patient factors and chart note communication. *Health Qual Life Outcomes.* 2015;13:161.
4. Copay AG, Glassman SD, Subach BR, Berven S, Schuler TC, Carreon LY. Minimum clinically important difference in lumbar spine surgery patients: a choice of methods using the Oswestry Disability Index, Medical Outcomes Study questionnaire Short Form 36, and pain scales. *Spine J.* 2008;8(6):968-974.
5. Lee JS, Hobden E, Stiell IG, Wells GA. Clinically important change in the visual analog scale after adequate pain control. *Acad Emerg Med.* 2003;10(10):1128-1130.
6. Tarlov AR, Ware Jr JE, Greenfield S, et al. The Medical Outcomes Study: an application of methods for monitoring the results of medical care. *JAMA.* 1989;262(7):925-930.
7. Ware Jr J, Kosinski M, Keller SD. A 12-Item Short-Form Health Survey: construction of scales and preliminary tests of reliability and validity. *Med Care.* 1996;34(3):220-233.
8. Hays RD, Sherbourne CD, Mazel RM. The rand 36-item health survey 1.0. *Health Econ.* 1993;2(3):217-227.
9. Cella D, Riley W, Stone A, et al. Patient-Reported Outcomes Measurement Information System (PROMIS) developed and tested its first wave of adult self-reported health outcome item banks: 2005–2008. *J Clin Epidemiol.* 2010;63(11):1179-1194.
10. Lauridsen HH, Hartvigsen J, Manniche C, Korsholm L, Grunnet-Nilsson N. Responsiveness and Minimal Clinically Important Difference for pain and disability instruments in low back pain patients. *BMC Musculoskelet Disord.* 2006;7:82.
11. Vernon H, Mior S. The Neck Disability Index: a study of reliability and validity. *J Manipulative Physiol Ther.* 1991;14(7):409-415.
12. Young BA, Walker MJ, Strunce JB, Boyles RE, Whitman JM, Childs JD. Responsiveness of the Neck Disability Index in patients with mechanical neck disorders. *Spine J.* 2009;9(10):802-808.
13. Button KS, Kounali D, Thomas L, et al. Minimal clinically important difference on the Beck Depression Inventory-II according to the patient's perspective. *Psychol Med.* 2015;45(15):3269-3279.
14. Jensen MP, Karoly P, Braver S. The measurement of clinical pain intensity: a comparison of six methods. *Pain.* 1986;27(1):117-126.
15. Grevitt M, Khazim R, Webb J, Mulholland R, Shepperd J. The Short Form-36 health survey questionnaire in spine surgery. *J Bone Joint Surg Br.* 1997;79(1):48-52.
16. Guilfoyle MR, Seeley H, Laing RJ. The Short Form 36 health survey in spine disease–validation against condition-specific measures. *Br J Neurosurg.* 2009;23(4):401-405.
17. Kapetanakis S, Gkasdaris GG, Thomaidis T, Charitoudis G, Nastoulis E, Givissis P. Postoperative evaluation of Health-Related Quality-of-Life (HRQoL) of patients with lumbar degenerative spondylolisthesis after instrumented Posterolateral Fusion (PLF): a prospective study with a 2-year follow-up. *Open Orthop J.* 2017;11:1423-1431.
18. Boden SH, Farley KX, Campbell C, et al. Rational selection of patient-reported outcomes measures in lumbar spine surgery patients. *Int J Spine Surg.* 2020;14(3):347-354.
19. Boody BS, Bhatt S, Mazmudar AS, Hsu WK, Rothrock NE, Patel AA. Validation of Patient-Reported Outcomes Measurement Information System (PROMIS) computerized adaptive tests in cervical spine surgery. *J Neurosurg Spine.* 2018;28(3):268-279.
20. Patel AA, Dodwad S-NM, Boody BS, et al. Validation of Patient Reported Outcomes Measurement Information System (PROMIS) computer adaptive tests (CATs) in the surgical treatment of lumbar spinal stenosis. *Spine (Phila Pa 1976).* 2018;43(21):1521-1528.
21. Roland M, Fairbank J. The Roland–Morris disability questionnaire and the Oswestry disability questionnaire. *Spine (Phila Pa 1976).* 2000;25(24):3115-3124.
22. Carreon LY, Glassman SD, Campbell MJ, Anderson PA. Neck Disability Index, Short Form-36 physical component summary, and pain scales for neck and arm pain: the minimum clinically important difference and substantial clinical benefit after cervical spine fusion. *Spine J.* 2010;10(6):469-474.
23. Chaichana KL, Mukherjee D, Adogwa O, Cheng JS, McGirt MJ. Correlation of preoperative depression and somatic perception scales with postoperative disability and quality of life after lumbar discectomy. *J Neurosurg Spine.* 2011;14(2):261-267.
24. Pakarinen M, Vanhanen S, Sinikallio S, et al. Depressive burden is associated with a poorer surgical outcome among lumbar spinal stenosis patients: a 5-year follow-up study. *Spine J.* 2014;14(10):2392-2396.
25. Al Amer HS, Alanazi F, Eldesoky M, et al. Cross-cultural adaptation and psychometric testing of the Arabic version of the Modified Oswestry Low Back Pain Disability Questionnaire. *PLoS One.* 2020;15(4):e0231382.
26. Schwartz CE, Stark RB, Balasuberamaniam P, Shrikumar M, Wasim A, Finkelstein JA. Responsiveness of standard spine outcome tools: do they measure up? *J Neurosurg Spine.* 2020;33(1):106-113.

Index

Page numbers followed by *b, t,* and *f* indicate boxes, tables, and figures, respectively.